Management of Compressive Neuropathies of the Upper Extremity

Guest Editor

ASIF M. ILYAS, MD

ORTHOPEDIC CLINICS OF NORTH AMERICA

www.orthopedic.theclinics.com

October 2012 • Volume 43 • Number 4

SAUNDERS an imprint of ELSEVIER, Inc.

W.B. SAUNDERS COMPANY
A Division of Elsevier Inc.

1600 John F. Kennedy Blvd. • Suite 1800 • Philadelphia, PA 19103-2899.

http://www.orthopedic.theclinics.com

ORTHOPEDIC CLINICS OF NORTH AMERICA Volume 43, Number 4
October 2012 ISSN 0030-5898, ISBN-13: 978-1-4557-5846-3

Editor: David Parsons

Orthopedic Clinics of North America (ISSN 0030-5898) is published quarterly by Elsevier Inc., 360 Park Avenue South, New York, NY 10010-1710. Months of issue are January, April, July, and October. Business and Editorial Offices: 1600 John F. Kennedy Blvd., Suite 1800, Philadelphia, PA 19103-2899. Customer Service Office: 3251 Riverport Lane, Maryland Heights, MO 63043. Periodicals postage paid at New York, NY and additional mailing offices. Subscription prices are $293.00 per year for (US individuals), $554.00 per year for (US institutions), $347.00 per year (Canadian individuals), $664.00 per year (Canadian institutions), $427.00 per year (international individuals), $664.00 per year (international institutions), $144.00 per year (US students), $208.00 per year (Canadian and international students). Foreign air speed delivery is included in all *Clinics* subscription prices. All prices are subject to change without notice. **POSTMASTER:** Send change of address to *Orthopedic Clinics of North America*, **Elsevier Health Sciences Division, Subscription Customer Service, 3251 Riverport Lane, Maryland Heights, MO 63043. Customer Service (orders, claims, online, change of address): Elsevier Health Sciences Division, Subscription Customer Service, 3251 Riverport Lane, Maryland Heights, MO 63043. Tel: 1-800-654-2452 (U.S. and Canada); 314-447-8871 (outside U.S. and Canada). Fax: 314-447-8029. E-mail: journalscustomerservice-usa@elsevier. com (for print support); journalsonlinesupport-usa@elsevier.com (for online support).**

Reprints. For copies of 100 or more, of articles in this publication, please contact the Commercial Reprints Department, Elsevier Inc., 360 Park Avenue South, New York, NY 10010-1710. Tel.: 212-633-3812; Fax: 212-462-1935; E-mail: reprints@elsevier. com.

Orthopedic Clinics of North America is covered in *MEDLINE/PubMed* (*Index Medicus*), *Cinahl, Excerpta Medica,* and *Cumulative Index to Nursing and Allied Health Literature.*

Printed and bound by CPI Group (UK) Ltd, Croydon, CR0 4YY

Transferred to digital print 2012

Contributors

GUEST EDITOR

ASIF M. ILYAS, MD
Program Director of Hand & Upper Extremity Surgery - Rothman Institute, Associate Professor of Orthopaedic Surgery - Thomas Jefferson University, Philadelphia, Pennsylvania

AUTHORS

ABDO BACHOURA, MD
The Philadelphia Hand Center, Philadelphia, Pennsylvania

RANDIP R. BINDRA, MD
Professor, Department of Orthopaedic Surgery and Rehabilitation, Loyola University Medical Center, Maywood, Illinois

THOMAS CHERIYAN, MD
Research Fellow, Orthopaedic Hand Service, Massachusetts General Hospital, Boston, Massachusetts

DIMITRIOS CHRISTOFOROU, MD
Hand Fellow, Orthopaedic Hand Service, Massachusetts General Hospital, Boston, Massachusetts

MITCHELL FREEDMAN, DO
Rothman Institute, Associate Professor, Thomas Jefferson University Hospital, Philadelphia

HILTON P. GOTTSCHALK, MD
Central Texas Pediatric Orthopedics, Austin, Texas

GARETT HELBER, DO
Resident, Physical Medicine and Rehabilitation, Thomas Jefferson University Hospital, Philadelphia

ASIF M. ILYAS, MD
Program Director, Hand & Upper Extremity Surgery, Rothman Institute; Associate Professor of Orthopaedic Surgery, Thomas Jefferson University, Philadelphia, Pennsylvania

SIDNEY M. JACOBY, MD
The Philadelphia Hand Center; Department of Orthopaedic Surgery, Thomas Jefferson University Hospital, Philadelphia, Pennsylvania

JIA-WEI KEVIN KO, MD
Assistant Professor, Department of Orthopedics, Oregon Health and Science University, Portland, Oregon

LEO T. KROONEN, MD
Assistant Professor, Uniformed Services University of Health Sciences, Hand & Microvascular Surgery, Department of Orthopaedic Surgery, Naval Medical Center San Diego, San Diego, California

CHARLES F. LEINBERRY Jr, MD
Hand & Upper Extremity Surgeon, Rothman Institute, Associate Professor of Orthopaedic Surgery, Thomas Jefferson University, Philadelphia, Pennsylvania

JONAS L. MATZON, MD
Assistant Professor, Orthopaedic Surgery, Rothman Institute, Thomas Jefferson University, Philadelphia, Pennsylvania

DOMINIC J. MINTALUCCI, MD
Fellow, Hand Surgery, Jefferson Medical College, Philadelphia, Pennsylvania

ADAM J. MIRARCHI, MD
Orthopedic Resident, Department of Orthopedics, Oregon Health and Science University, Portland, Oregon

CHAITANYA S. MUDGAL, MD
Interim Chief, Program Director, Orthopaedic Hand Service, Massachusetts General Hospital, Boston, Massachusetts

NASH H. NAAM, MD
Clinical Professor, Plastic and Reconstructive Surgery, Southern Illinois Hand Center, Southern Illinois University, Effingham, Illinois

KATE NELLANS, MD, MPH
Department of Orthopaedic Surgery, New York Presbyterian Hospital, Columbia University, New York, New York

SAJJAN NEMANI, MD
Department of Neurology, Southern Illinois Hand Center, Effingham, Illinois

VALENTIN NEUHAUS, MD
Research Fellow, Orthopaedic Hand Service, Massachusetts General Hospital, Boston, Massachusetts

GENGHIS E. NIVER, MD
Fellow, Hand and Upper Extremity Surgery, Rothman Institute, Thomas Jefferson University, Philadelphia, Pennsylvania

MEREDITH OSTERMAN, MD
Resident, Orthopaedic Surgery, Thomas Jefferson University, Philadelphia, Pennsylvania

SAMUEL P. POPINCHALK, MD
Resident, Department of Orthopaedic Surgery and Sports Medicine, Temple University, Philadelphia, Pennsylvania

JASON POTHAST, MD
Resident, Physical Medicine and Rehabilitation, Thomas Jefferson University Hospital, Philadelphia

ALYSSA A. SCHAFFER, MD
Assistant Professor, Department of Orthopaedic Surgery and Sports Medicine, Temple University, Philadelphia, Pennsylvania

LIANE SHER, MD
Magee Rehabilitation Hospital, Assistant Professor, Thomas Jefferson University Hospital, Philadelphia

JEREMY SIMON, MD
Clinical Instructor, Physical Medicine, Rothman Institute, Thomas Jefferson University Hospital, Philadelphia

PETER TANG, MD, MPH
Department of Orthopaedic Surgery, Assistant Professor of Clinical Orthopedic Surgery, New York Presbyterian Hospital, Columbia University, New York, New York

RICK TOSTI, MD
Resident, Orthopaedic Surgery, Temple University Hospital, Philadelphia, Pennsylvania

ALICIA WORDEN, MD
Resident, Orthopaedic Surgery, Saint Louis University, St Louis, Missouri

T.G. SHAHWAN, MD
Resident, Physical Medicine and Rehabilitation, Thomas Jefferson University, Malvern, Philadelphia

Contents

innervation to most of the volar forearm musculature and, importantly, to m ost of thenar musculature. The main goal of median nerve reconstructive procedures is to restore thumb opposition. There are a variety of transfers that can achieve this goal but tendon transfers must recreate thumb opposition, which involves 3 basics movements: thumb abduction, flexion, and pronation. Many tendon transfers exist and the choice of tendon transfer should be tailored to the patient's needs.

Acute carpal tunnel syndrome is characterized by rapid onset of median neuropathy caused by sudden increases in carpal tunnel pressures, which leads to ischemia of the median nerve. The most common cause is traumatic injury, although atraumatic sources should also be recognized. Patients generally complain of pain, lose two-point discrimination, and may demonstrate elevated compartment pressure on measurement. Prompt recognition and surgical decompression are imperative to spare median nerve viability.

Ulnar tunnel syndrome could be broadly defined as a compressive neuropathy of the ulnar nerve at the level of the wrist. The ulnar tunnel, or Guyon's canal, has a complex and variable anatomy. Various factors may precipitate the onset of ulnar tunnel syndrome. Patient presentation depends on the anatomic zone of ulnar nerve compression: zone I compression, motor and sensory signs and symptoms; zone II compression, isolated motor deficits; and zone III compression; purely sensory deficits. Conservative treatment such as activity modification may be helpful, but often, surgical exploration of the ulnar tunnel with subsequent ulnar nerve decompression is indicated.

Compression of the ulnar nerve at the elbow, or cubital tunnel syndrome, is the second most common peripheral nerve compression syndrome in the upper extremity. Diagnosis is made through a good history and physical examination. Electrodiagnostic testing can confirm the diagnosis and severity of injury to the nerve. Surgical intervention is indicated when nonoperative treatment does not relieve the symptoms. There is currently no consensus on the best surgical treatment of cubital tunnel syndrome. However, the only randomized prospective studies to compare treatment options to date indicate that simple decompression and anterior transposition yield comparable results.

Failure after ulnar nerve decompression at the elbow can be defined as either no change in the patient's symptoms or an initial improvement with recurrence, making the patient history essential in the work-up. Failure may be due to diagnostic, technical, or biologic factors. Technical errors and the development of perineural fibrosis necessitate revision surgery, while nerve damage due to chronic severe compression should be observed. We do not believe any one procedure is superior in the revision setting as long as a complete decompression is achieved with a compression free, stable transposition of the surgeon's choice.

Ulnar nerve palsy results in significant loss of sensation and profound weakness, leading to a dysfunctional hand. Typical clinical findings include loss of key pinch, clawing, loss of normal flexion sequence of the digits, loss of the metacarpal arch, and abduction of the small finger. Further deficits in hand/wrist function are seen in high-level ulnar nerve palsy, including loss of ring- and small-finger distal interphalangeal flexion, decreased wrist flexion, and loss of dorsal sensory innervation. This article reviews the clinical findings seen in low and high ulnar nerve palsies, and reviews surgical options for correcting certain motor and sensory deficits.

Ulnar nerve dysfunction is a well-recognized phenomenon following distal humerus fractures. Its fixed anatomic position predisposes the nerve to injury. Injury can occur at the time of injury, during closed-fracture manipulation, intraoperatively during fracture fixation (when it is routinely identified), or during fracture healing. Intraoperative management varies widely and can include in situ decompression or anterior transposition. This article reviews the literature and presents 24 patient cases. A 38% incidence of late ulnar neuropathy following open reduction and internal fixation is identified. There is no statistical difference between an in situ release and all anterior transpositions, except for submuscular.

During pregnancy, hormonal fluctuations, fluid shifts, and musculoskeletal changes predispose women to carpal tunnel syndrome. While the clinical presentation is similar to other patients, the history obtained must include information regarding the pregnancy itself. Currently, the indication for electrodiagnostic testing is not clearly defined. Given that symptoms often improve with conservative treatment and abate after delivery, EMG/NCV testing can often be avoided. However, if symptoms are severe or persist, carpal tunnel release is indicated and is considered a safe procedure for both mother and fetus.

Carpal tunnel syndrome is a common condition and is a well-recognized phenomenon following a distal radius fracture. The treating surgeon should be vigilant in noticing the signs and symptoms. If acute carpal tunnel syndrome is noted, then surgical release of the carpal tunnel and fracture fixation should be performed urgently. If early carpal tunnel syndrome findings are noted during distal radius fracture management, all potential causes should be evaluated. Delayed carpal tunnel syndrome presenting after a distal radius fracture has healed is best managed in standard fashion. There is no role for prophylactic carpal tunnel release at the time of distal radius fixation in a patient who is asymptomatic.

Nash H. Naam and Sajjan Nemani

Radial tunnel syndrome is a pain syndrome resulting from compression of the posterior interosseous nerve at the proximal forearm. It has no specific radiologic or electrodiagnostic findings. Treatment should be started conservatively; if not successful, surgical treatment is indicated. The posterior interosseous nerve may be explored through dorsal or anterior approaches. All the potential sites of entrapment should be released, including complete release of the superficial head of the supinator muscle. Surgical treatment is generally successful, but patients who have associated lateral epicondylitis or those who are involved in workers' compensation claims have less successful outcomes.

ORTHOPEDIC CLINICS OF NORTH AMERICA

Preface

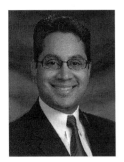

Asif M. Ilyas, MD
Guest Editor

Compressive neuropathies are among the most common pathologies of the upper extremity facing Orthopaedists. The most common compressive neuropathies include carpal tunnel syndrome, cubital tunnel syndrome, and radial tunnel syndrome. These lesions can occur spontaneously, secondary to certain activities, as a sequelae of medicalco-morbidities, and following trauma. With the help of an exceptional group of authors, this issue provides a practical review of physical examination findings, electrodiagnostic evaluations, and treatment options. In addition, we have highlighted the management of median andulnar neuropathies following distal radius and distal humerus fractures, respectively. Lastly, a detailed review of the management of late neuropathies is also provided.

Asif M. Ilyas, MD
Rothman Institute
Thomas Jefferson University Hospital
925 Chestnut Street
Philadelphia, PA 19107, USA

E-mail address:
asif.ilyas@rothmaninstitute.com

Orthop Clin N Am 43 (2012) xi
http://dx.doi.org/10.1016/j.ocl.2012.08.011

Electrodiagnostic Evaluation of Compressive Nerve Injuries of the Upper Extremities

Mitchell Freedman, DO[a],*, Garett Helber, DO[b],
Jason Pothast, MD[b], T.G. Shahwan, MD[c],
Jeremy Simon, MD[d], Liane Sher, MD[e]

KEYWORDS

- Electromyography • Nerve conduction studies • Compressive nerve injuries • Prognosis
- Wallerian degeneration • Neuropraxia • Axonotmesis • Neurotmesis

KEY POINTS

- Electromyography (EMG) and nerve conduction studies are diagnostic tools that evaluate the physiologic function of the peripheral nervous system, including the anterior horn cell, nerve roots, brachial plexus, peripheral nerves, neuromuscular junction, and muscle.
- This article reviews the common compressive nerve lesions of the upper extremity as well as the utility of EMG/nerve conduction velocity in assisting with diagnosis, localization, timing, severity, and prognosis for recovery.

Electromyography and nerve conduction studies (EMG/NCS) are diagnostic tools that evaluate the physiologic function of the peripheral nervous system, including the anterior horn cell, nerve roots, brachial plexus, peripheral nerves, neuromuscular junction, and muscle. It is guided by and interpreted in light of a thorough neuromuscular evaluation. This article reviews the common compressive nerve lesions of the upper extremity as well as the utility of EMG/nerve conduction velocity (NCV) in assisting with diagnosis, localization, timing, severity, and prognosis for recovery.

CLASSIFICATION OF PERIPHERAL NERVE LESIONS

The peripheral nerve is made up of the internal axon and the external myelin sheath as well as the surrounding stroma. The major classification system for nerve injuries describe the injury based on the architecture of the injury to these structures. The Seddon classification[1] divides nerve lesions into the following groupings: neuropraxia, axonotmesis, and neurotmesis.

Neuropraxia represents damage to the myelin. There is no damage to the axon, and therefore there is no Wallerian degeneration. This is the mildest form of lesion, and symptoms may resolve within seconds to up to 3 to 6 months.[2] Axonotmesis occurs as a result of damage to the axon and myelin, but the surrounding Schwann tubes, endoneurium, and perineurium are partially or fully intact. However, axonotmesis does result in Wallerian degeneration of the axon. Wallerian degeneration begins at about 3 days and is completed over 11 days in the sensory fibers and over

[a] Rothman Institute, Thomas Jefferson University Hospital, 925 Chestnut Street, Philadelphia, PA 19107, USA;
[b] Physical Medicine and Rehabilitation, Thomas Jefferson University Hospital, 10th and Chestnut Street, Philadelphia, PA 19107, USA; [c] Physical Medicine and Rehabilitation, Thomas Jefferson University, 414 Paoli Pike, Malvern, PA 19355, USA; [d] Physical Medicine, Rothman Institute, Thomas Jefferson University Hospital, 925 Chestnut Street, Philadelphia, PA 19107, USA; [e] Magee Rehabilitation Hospital, Thomas Jefferson University Hospital, 6 Franklin Plaza, Philadelphia, PA 19102, USA
* Corresponding author.
E-mail address: lm5656@comcast.net

Orthop Clin N Am 43 (2012) 409–416
http://dx.doi.org/10.1016/j.ocl.2012.07.010

orthopedic.theclinics.com

9 days in the motor fibers because of the earlier failure of the neuromuscular junction. Thus, EMG/NCV may not be able to distinguish between neuropraxia and axonotmesis until Wallerian degeneration has had time to occur. Recovery begins via sprouting from the tip of the peripheral motor nerve within 1 week. Recovery via direct regrowth involving the motor and sensory aspect of the nerve is variable, but occurs at an average of 1 mm/d. However the rate of regrowth is decreased in cases with more proximal or severe lesions, older patients, and cases with significant scar tissue.

In axonotmesis, the axon and myelin are injured, but the surrounding Schwann tubes, endoneurium, and perineurium are partially or fully intact. In contrast, with neurotmesis, there is damage to the axon and myelin, and the architecture of the endoneurial tube is completely disrupted, which makes regrowth less likely. EMG/NCV is not typically able to distinguish between severe axonotmesis and neurotmesis.[3–5]

Unlike motor function recovery, sensory function does not recover via sprouting. There is recovery via axonal regeneration. There may also be redistribution of sensory nerve coverage after an axonal injury, which results in the remaining uninjured fibers supplying cutaneous sensation to a larger area than was supplied before the injury.[5,6]

TERMS OF EMG/NCV

Electromyography evaluates individual muscles at rest as well as with submaximal and maximal voluntary muscle contractions. At rest, the muscle is evaluated with 5 to 30 needle passes in different quadrants at each site. Each time the needle electrode is moved, there is a release of self-limited electrical activity. This activity is called insertional activity and may be increased when there is damage to the axon. If the muscle is fibrotic, then the insertional activity is decreased. Spontaneous abnormal electrical potentials that result from axonal damage are called positive waves and fibrillations. These abnormal electrical potentials may be seen as early as 7 to 10 days after injury, but may not be seen for 3 to 4 weeks. The number of these potentials does not correlate with the severity of the injury. Fibrillations are generally seen more acutely and tend to disappear over the next year. Chronic findings are identified by small fibrillations or complex repetitive discharges. Submaximal contraction looks at the contraction of the individual motor units. If there is subacute to chronic damage to the nerve, polyphasic potentials are seen. These potentials are wave forms with 5 or more phases that form as a result of collateral nerve sprouting, remyelination,

and reinnervation. Over time, the polyphasic activity resolves and maximal contraction reveals large amplitude potential as a result of electrical summation of the multiple sprouts that have remyelinated. If there is enough damage, the remaining individual neurons and the muscle fibers that they innervate will fire at an increased rate, because there are few nerve fibers innervating the muscle. This is called decreased recruitment and may be a result of repetitive firing of the individual motor units; this may well correlate with clinical weakness. In myelinopathy, the only finding on EMG may be decreased or absent firing of the motor units because of conduction block.[7]

NCS are performed on motor and sensory nerves. The temperature in the upper extremity should be at least 32° or the distal latency and conduction velocity may be artificially slow. The time that it takes the nerve to conduct from the point of stimulation to the active electrode over the muscle or to another electrode over the sensory nerve is called the distal latency. The electrical potential that is created with stimulation of the motor nerve is the compound muscle action potential (CMAP), whereas the sensory potential is called the compound sensory nerve action potential (SNAP). Normal values are based on the results in a normal population, but may also be derived by comparing the nerve in question to another peripheral nerve or the same contralateral nerve. The distal latency may be abnormal as a result of myelinopathy more than axonopathy, unless the axonal pathology is severe. Conduction velocity represents the speed of electrical conduction in the nerve. Severe slowing of the NCV is usually the result of myelinopathy, and mild NCV slowing is more attributed to axonopathy. Prolonged distal latency and slow conduction velocity usually do not result in clinical signs seen on physical examination.

In cases of myelinopathy, the electrical impulses travel at divergent speeds in the individual axons across a lesion, resulting in temporal dispersion when the wave form that is achieved with stimulation proximal to the lesion is 20% to 30% longer than the wave form that results from stimulation of the nerve distal to the lesion. This may or may not result in clinical signs seen on physical examination. Conduction block is seen when all or a portion of the impulses are not conducted across the lesion. Proximal stimulation results in an action potential that will achieve an amplitude more than 20% smaller than the potential evoked with stimulation distal to the conduction block.

In cases of axonopathy, the amplitude of the evoked response proximal and distal to the lesion will also be diminished secondary to Wallerian degeneration. The degree of diminution of the amplitude is relative to the unaffected side or accepted "norm" comparable to the severity of the injury. It does result in changes, which will be seen on physical examination. Conduction block and temporal dispersion are findings that assist in localization of the lesion in myelinopathy. NCV is not as useful in localizing the lesion with axonopathy, because axonal lesions result in diminished amplitude proximal and distal to the lesion. In axonopathy, the EMG is used to localize the lesion based on muscles that are abnormal.

PITFALLS OF EMG/NCV

EMG/NCV is not a perfect test, and interpretation must be formulated and interpreted in the light of the clinical evaluation. This test does not determine the exact cause of the neurologic lesion. There are technical and operator-dependent errors, which may lead to incorrect conclusions. Correct wave form evaluation is subjective and operator dependent. Normal variations in the composition of fascicles in nerve roots and the peripheral nerves may result in different patterns of muscle innervation may confuse the localization of the lesion on EMG as well as the physical examination.

Only a portion of the muscle is evaluated when performing the EMG, and the muscle may look normal when it is not normal. If the study is performed too early, sufficient time may not have passed to evaluate whether or not muscle abnormalities are present. Later in the course of an injury, the signs of fibrillations and positive waves may disappear, to be replaced by the more chronic findings of polyphasicity and large amplitude potentials on needle testing. Chronic nerve injury may be difficult to identify on EMG. As patients age, a percentage of muscle fibers normally develop polyphasic potentials, which can lead to false-positive conclusions. Positive waves and fibrillations may be seen in myopathy as well as with direct trauma or injections into the muscle.

In more acute lesions with mixed axonopathy and myelinopathy, prognostication on NCS findings is unreliable. In certain nerves, it may not be feasible to stimulate the nerve proximal and distal to the injury and establish whether or not there is a myelinopathy. The number of positive waves and fibrillations do not correlate with the severity of the injury. If there is no evidence of myelinopathy, the amplitude of the evoked response can be used to understand the degree of axonal lesion in the acute phase. If the amplitude of the evoked response on the affected side is greater than 30% of the intact contralateral nerve, the prognosis for recovery is good. If the amplitude is between 10%

and 30% of the contralateral nerve, the prognosis is fair, and it is poor if the amplitude is less than 10% of the other side.[8] In the subacute to chronic phase, sprouting and regrowth result in increased amplitude of the evoked motor response, and it can no longer be used for prognostication.

ANATOMY

In the cervical spine, there are 8 cervical nerve roots that exit from their respective foramen, except for C8, which exits from the C7-T1 foramen. The dorsal root ganglion of the sensory nerve root generally resides in the neural foramen. The brachial plexus is the continuation of the nerves as they extend distally after exiting the neural foramen from the cervical spine. It is a network of peripheral nerves comprised of the ventral rami of C5 through T1 that travel distally and divide into trunks, divisions, cords, and branches. Entrapment or compression of the exiting spinal nerve root may occur by a cervical disc herniation, hypertrophy of the uncovertebral joints of Lushka, facet arthropathy, and combinations of these processes. The brachial plexus may be injured due to a mass lesion, a penetrating wound, autoimmune/microvascular phenomenon (ie, neuralgic amyotrophy of Parsonage-Turner) or a stretch injury.

Suprascapular Nerve

The suprascapular nerve originates from the upper trunk of the brachial plexus and is composed of the C5 and C6 nerve roots. The nerve crosses the posterior triangle of the neck, travels beneath the trapezius, dives through the suprascapular notch under the transverse scapular ligament, and enters the suprascapular fossa, where it innervates the supraspinatus muscle. The nerve then wraps around the spinoglenoid notch under the spinoglenoid ligament to innervate the infraspinatus muscle. Entrapment of the suprascapular nerve at the suprascapular notch results in denervation of the supraspinatus and infraspinatus muscles. Because the scapula and shoulder are mobile, tethering of the nerve may occur under the transverse scapular ligament,[9] especially in repetitive overhead activities. Scapular fractures, direct trauma due to heavy backpacks, and ganglion cysts secondary to superior and posterior labral tears may also cause compression of the nerve.[10] Compression of the suprascapular nerve by paralabral or ganglion cysts at the spinoglenoid notch results in denervation of the infraspinatus muscle. Moreover, tightening the spinoglenoid ligament by repetitive overhead activities can also compress the nerve at this location.[11]

Motor nerve conductions are performed by stimulating at Erb point and recording at the supraspinatus and infraspinatus with a superficial or intramuscular needle electrode. Intramuscular recording electrodes can only record from nearby fibers. However, surface electrode recording is unreliable because of volume conduction distortion from the bulky nature of the overlying trapezius muscle. In acute axonal lesions, EMG will reveal positive waves and fibrillations in the infraspinatus if the lesion is at the spinoglenoid notch, whereas both the supraspinatus and infraspinatus will be abnormal if the lesion is at the suprascapular notch. EMG may normalize in chronic conditions. With abnormalities in the infraspinatus, one must carry out additional needle examination to ensure no evidence of a C5 radiculopathy, C6 radiculopathy, or upper trunk brachial plexopathy.

Axillary Nerve

The axillary nerve originates from the upper trunk and posterior cord of the brachial plexus, receiving innervations from the C5 and C6 nerve roots. The nerve passes posterior to the axillary artery, inferior to the glenohumeral surface, and enters the quadrilateral space, whose borders include the teres minor muscle superiorly, teres major muscle inferiorly, long of the triceps brachii muscle medially, and the proximal humerus laterally. After exiting the quadrilateral space, the axillary nerve divides into an anterior branch, which innervates the middle and anterior fibers of the deltoid muscle, and a posterior branch, which innervates teres minor, the deltoid muscle's posterior fibers, and sensation via the upper lateral cutaneous nerve of the arm. Most causes of axillary neuropathies are traumatic in nature. However, compression of the axillary nerve can occur as it exits posteriorly through the quadrilateral space, commonly referred to as quadrilateral space syndrome. Compression at this site may be caused by repetitive overhead activities, hypertrophy of the muscles bordering the quadrilateral space, paralabral cysts, or fibrous bands within the space.[12]

Motor nerve conductions are performed by stimulation at Erb point with surface electrode recording from the deltoid muscle. Unfortunately, stimulation at Erb point not only stimulates the axillary nerve but also stimulates the entire brachial plexus and may result in an unreliable response secondary to volume conduction from other nearby musculature. One must compare CMAPs between both sides as there can be considerable variability in the latencies and amplitudes. EMG reveals positive waves and fibrillations in the deltoid and/or teres minor muscles with acute axonal lesions.

Radial Nerve

The radial nerve originates from the posterior cord and all 3 trunks of the brachial plexus, receiving innervations from the C5-T1 nerve roots. In the axillary region, the nerve gives branches to the 3 heads of the triceps muscle. The radial nerve dives posterolaterally between the lateral and medial heads of the triceps brachii muscle and wraps around the midshaft of the humerus in the spiral groove. At the lateral margin of the humerus, radial nerve pierces the lateral intermuscular septum, innervates the brachioradialis and possibly the brachialis, and passes between those muscles. The extensor carpi radialis longus (ECRL) is innervated proximal to the lateral epicondyle. The extensor carpi radialis brevis (ECRB) is next innervated by the main trunk of the radial nerve or the superficial radial nerve and or/the posterior interosseous nerve. At the level of the radiocapitellar joint, the posterior interosseous nerve enters the radial tunnel; dives under the arcade of Frohse, a fibrous arch formed by the proximal portion of the supinator muscle; and enters the supinator muscle between the humeral and ulnar origins. After exiting from the supinator muscle, the posterior interosseous nerve splits into multiple smaller branches to innervate the extensor muscles of the forearm and terminates into the extensor indicis proprius (EIP) muscle. The superficial radial nerve splits from the main trunk of the radial nerve proximal to the supinator and continues distally underneath the brachioradialis muscle, becomes superficial, and crosses the dorsolateral wrist to supply cutaneous sensation to a thenar portion of the dorsal hand.[13]

The radial nerve is infrequently compressed by crutches or poor sleep posture in the axilla, resulting in weakness of all of the radial musculature. It is more frequently compressed in the medial upper arm, near the spiral groove or the distal lateral upper arm. Direct injury or traction occur most commonly following fractures of the humerus. Compression may also occur with lying for a prolonged period over the lateral arm (ie, Saturday night palsy), prolonged tourniquet application, or by a hypertrophied triceps muscle. Similarly, injury to the radial nerve also frequently occurs at the elbow and proximal forearm. Posterior interosseous neuropathy may be compressed by 5 structures: fibrous bands arising from the brachioradialis, branches of the radial recurrent artery, the leading edge of the ECRB, the proximal edge of the supinator (the arcade of Frohse), and the distal edge of the supinator[14]; this would spare the ECRL and result in radial deviation of the wrist with muscle testing. External compression of the superficial radial nerve can occur at the wrist via handcuffs, jewelry, and casts.

CMAPs can be obtained with surface recording electrodes over the EIP while stimulating below the elbow, above the elbow, and in the axilla. Radial nerve motor conduction studies are technically challenging and can be difficult to accurately elicit a true response because of the size of the EIP and its close proximity to other radial innervated muscles. EMG will reveal abnormalities in the triceps and distal radial musculature with a proximal lesion at the axilla. EMG will reveal sparing of the triceps, but abnormalities will exist in the distal radial innervated musculature if the injury is at the level of the spiral groove. Axonal lesion at the level of the axilla and spiral groove affects the CMAP recorded from the EIP as well as the SNAP recorded from the superficial radial sensory nerve. Compression within the radial tunnel affects only the posterior interosseous nerve and spares the triceps and the ECRL as well as the superficial radial sensory nerve. A lesion at this location will affect only the radial CMAP, not the SNAP of the superficial radial sensory nerve. Localization of the lesion can be complex in incomplete lesions as needle examination may show abnormalities in a patchy distribution of muscles.

Ulnar Nerve

The ulnar nerve is derived from the C8 and T1 nerve roots, which form the lower trunk of the brachial plexus that is formed after passing between the medial and anterior scalene muscles. The anterior division of the lower trunk gives rise to the medial cord on the lateral wall of the axilla. This nerve runs medial and posterior to the axillary vessels in the axilla and medial to the brachial artery in the upper arm. The ulnar nerve descends in a groove between coracobrachialis laterally and the triceps posteriorly before piercing through the intermuscular septum and entering the posterior compartment of the arm and travels along the medial head of the triceps and passes into the ulnar (retrocondylar) groove behind the medial epicondyle. As the nerve emerges from the groove, it passes under the aponeurotic arch of the flexor carpi ulnaris (FCU) muscle (humeroulnar arcade) formed from the attachment of the muscle to the medial epicondyle and the olecranon. The nerve then resides in the cubital tunnel, which has a roof composed of the aponeurotic arch and the FCU, and a floor composed of the medial ligaments of the elbow and the FCU. The nerve then courses between muscle layers of the FCU before passing deep to the FCU and anterior to the flexor digitorum profundus (FDP) as it descends into the forearm. The FCU receives variable dual innervation from the median nerve as well as the ulnar nerve. Proximal to the wrist, the ulnar nerve gives off a sensory palmar branch, which innervates the hypothenar eminence, and the dorsal ulnar cutaneous nerve (DUC), a sensory nerve which innervates the dorsal one and a half digital branches to the fourth and fifth digits. At the wrist, the nerve passes between the pisiform bone and the hook of the hamate through Guyon canal where it divides into the superficial and deep terminal branches within the canal. Compression injury to the ulnar nerve in the axilla and upper arm is uncommon. This damage may occur from external compression from the use of crutches,[15] tourniquet,[16] and pressure during sleep. The arcade of Struthers is a septum of variable thickness, which extends from the medial intermuscular septum from the upper surface of the triceps between 3 and 6 cm proximal to the medial epicondyle. It infrequently tethers the nerve to the triceps. The 2 major sites of ulnar neuropathies at the elbow are the retrocondylar groove and the humeroulnar arcade (cubital tunnel). Fractures or arthropathies of the elbow are the main causes, which may result in disfigurement of the elbow joint and predispose the ulnar nerve to compression.[17] Elbow flexion increases the potential for nerve damage due to narrowing of the cubital tunnel. Prolapse of the ulnar nerve out of the retrocondylar groove with elbow flexion also increases the nerve's susceptibility to external compression.

Chronic and repetitive external pressure on the ulnar nerve in the hand and wrist occurs over time. Bicycling is the best known cause of these neuropathies. There are 4 potential sites of injury to the ulnar nerve at this level. Type 1 involves the main trunk of the nerve at the entrance or within Guyon canal and results in sensory loss of the ulnar one and a half fingers and weakness of all ulnar intrinsic muscles. Type 2 involves the deep terminal (motor) branch of the ulnar nerve distal to Guyon canal; the sensory branch is spared while all ulnar intrinsics are weak. Type 3 involves the motor branch distal to the branches that innervate the hypothenar musculature. It is the most frequently seen lesion at the wrist and hand and involves the ulnar innervated lumbricals and interossei. Type 4 involves only the superficial terminal (sensory) branch producing only sensory loss.

The ulnar motor NCV across the elbow is the primary technique used to identify neuropathy at the elbow. An inching technique with sequential stimulations 1 to 2 cm apart across the elbow may be more sensitive and allow better localization of the lesion.[18] However, this does not evaluate the sensory aspect of the ulnar nerve across the elbow. The ulnar sensory nerve is better evaluated distally across the wrist. If the amplitude of the response, or in severe axonal lesions, the distal latency is abnormal, then further evaluation is warranted to determine whether or not the lesion is proximal to the wrist. If the lesion is proximal to the midforearm, then the amplitude of the DUC may be diminished or absent, whereas if the lesion is at the wrist, the DUC amplitude will be normal. If there is an axonal lesion below the elbow, then the EMG will be abnormal in the first dorsal interosseous (FDI) and adductor digiti minimi (ADM). In contrast, the FCU and the FDP are often spared if the lesion is at or below the elbow. If those muscles are also abnormal, then the lesion is definitively localized proximal to the wrist and is most likely at the elbow. It is important to evaluate the abductor pollicis brevis (APB) to rule out C8 radiculopathy or brachial plexopathy.[19]

An ulnar nerve lesion at the wrist is evaluated by stimulating the distal sensory nerve proximal to the wrist as well as by stimulating the motor nerve with the active electrode over the FDI and ADM. In a myelinopathy, stimulation of the ulnar sensory nerve in the palm results in a larger amplitude potential than the potential obtained with stimulation proximal to the wrist secondary to a conduction block. EMG of the FDI and ADM is performed to further evaluate whether or not there are signs of axonopathy.

Median Nerve

The median nerve is derived from the lateral and medial cords of the brachial plexus, which receive contributions from the superior, middle, and inferior trunks. The median nerve contains innervations from roots C6 through T1. The median nerve travels lateral to the brachial artery initially, but crosses medially in the proximal arm. It travels deep to the bicipital aponeurosis and passes between the 2 heads of the pronator teres. The median nerve usually gives branches to the pronator teres before passing through it and then branches to the rest of the proximal volar forearm musculature, except for the FCU and a portion of the FDP.

Before diving posterior and deep to the humeroulnar and radial origins of the flexor digitorum superficialis (FDS), the median nerve gives off the anterior interosseous nerve (AIN) that travels with it as it passes between the pronator heads and deep to the FDS. The median nerve continues into the forearm between the FDS and FDP, where it becomes superficial distally, gives off the palmar cutaneous branch, and then enters the carpal tunnel terminating into motor and sensory branches of the hand. The motor branches innervate the APB muscle, the

opponens pollicis, the superficial head of the flexor pollicis brevis, and the first and second lumbricals. The sensory fibers innervate the volar aspect of the thumb, index, middle, and radial half of the ring finger, including the distal palm and the dorsal, distal half of the aforementioned digits. Anatomic variations are not uncommon and often include a median-ulnar connection, known as the Martin-Gruber anastomosis and the Riche-Cannieu anastomosis. The AIN continues between the FDS and FDP and remains just volar to the interosseous membrane of the forearm. It variably innervates the thenar portion of the FDP, the flexor pollicis longus (FPL) alone or in conjunction with the median nerve, and is the sole innervation for the pronator quadrates (PQs).

Median nerve injury may occur at the axilla or upper arm via compression from crutches, fracture, trauma, sleep palsy, shoulder dislocation, tourniquet injury, or arteriovenous fistula. The ligament of Struthers, a fibrous band from the anteromedial aspect of the distal humerus to its medial epicondyle can compress the median nerve proximal to the elbow. Median neuropathy at the elbow can occur from local fractures or elbow dislocation or a mass; it is infrequently entrapped by the bicipital aponeurosis or the pronator teres (PT). The most common and distal entrapment of the median nerve is compression within the carpal tunnel. The AIN is infrequently compressed in isolation or in addition to the median nerve proper. Multiple sites of compression have been identified, including the brachialis fascia, bicipital bursa, PT, FCR, palmaris longus, accessory head of the FPL, aberrant radial artery, ulnar collateral vessels, and FDS.[20]

Electrodiagnostic studies have reported a sensitivity of 85% to 90% in carpal tunnel syndrome (CTS).[21] Sensory studies are considered more sensitive in diagnosing CTS because they are considered more susceptible to ischemia caused by mechanical compression. Comparison of the median sensory distal latency to another nerve in the ipsilateral limb, such as the distal radial or ulnar segment, not such as the radial or ulnar distal segment or the contralateral median sensory nerve, provides more accuracy than an absolute value; this serves to control for other factors such as age, temperature, systemic illnesses, gender, and hand size. A low-amplitude potential relative to the contralateral median nerve or to normal values indicates an axonal lesion. To prove that it is axonal, a stimulation distal to the carpal tunnel must be performed. If the amplitude of the response remains low, there is an axonal lesion, and if the amplitude of the evoked response increases significantly, then there is at least a partial myelinopathy. Distal latency in the motor nerve may be prolonged as well. There may be technical difficulties in obtaining an accurate wave form with stimulation of the motor or sensory nerve distal to the carpal tunnel, which make it difficult to establish whether or not there is an axonopathy or myelinopathy. EMG testing is optional, but may be helpful to investigate whether or not another neurologic lesion such as radiculopathy or plexopathy is present and to determine if there is an axonopathy involving the median nerve. Chronic compression of the nerve may result in a normal EMG, small positive waves, or large amplitude potentials.

True neurologic entrapment of the median nerve at the PT is an uncommon finding. Electrodiagnostic studies in PT entrapment are frequently found to be normal. In symptomatic patients, fewer than 50% of patients have electrodiagnostic findings.[22] Normal electrodiagnostic studies should not be used to exclude a pronator syndrome diagnosis in the proper clinical context. In cases where NCS abnormalities are demonstrable, slowing of the median motor conduction velocity across the elbow may be noted as well as a decrease in SNAP with stimulation of the nerve distally (if there is an axonal lesion). Conduction blocks are rare. Motor and sensory distal latencies and amplitudes are typically unaffected.[23] Proximal testing has not been typically performed in compressive entrapments by the lacertus fibrosus. When performed, the results are usually negative.[24] Distally, compression at the FDS may demonstrate slowed conduction velocities in the forearm, but distal sensory and motor latencies are present unless there is an associated CTS. EMG testing is typically more helpful in identifying acute proximal median nerve entrapments, if there is an axonal lesion, by identifying abnormal median innervated musculature distal to the injury.

Electrodiagnostic studies can also be helpful in diagnosing AIN compression. Diagnosis is generally made by the EMG with the PQ, FPL, or median branch of FDP demonstrating spontaneous activity such as positive waves or fibrillations. Standard nerve conductions involving the median nerve are generally normal, unless there is a concurrent carpal tunnel or more proximal median nerve lesion. Nerve conduction strategies to directly evaluate the AIN are used infrequently. The motor latency is typically abnormal or unobtainable. The CMAP is below normal and more often affected than latency.[25]

REFERENCES

1. Seddon HJ. Surgical disorders of the peripheral nerves. 2nd edition. New York: Churchill Livingstone; 1975. p. 21–3.

2. Stewart JD. Pathologic processes producing focal peripheral neuropathies. In: Stewart, editor. Focal peripheral neuropathies. 4th edition. West Vancouver (British Columbia): JBJ Publishing; 2010. p. 15–43.

3. Chaudry V, Cornblath DR. Wallerian degeration in human nerves: serial electrophysiological studies. Muscle Nerve 1992;15:687–93.

4. Sunderland S. The peripheral nerve trunk in relation to injury. a classification of nerve injury. In: Sunderland, editor. Nerves and nerve injuries. 2nd edition. New York: Churchill Livingstone; 1972. p. 127–37.

5. Robinson LR. Traumatic injury to peripheral nerves. Muscle Nerve 2000;23:863–73.

6. Speidel CC. Studies of living nerves: growth adjustments of cutaneous terminal arborization. J Comp Neurol 1942;76:57–73.

7. Daube JR, Rubin DI. Needle electromyography. Muscle Nerve 2009;39:244–70.

8. Zander Olsen P. Prediction of recovery in Bell's Palsy. Acta Neurol Scand 1975;52(S61):1–120.

9. Shapiro BE, Preston DC. Entrapment and compressive neuropathies. Med Clin North Am 2009;93(2): 285–315.

10. Bencardino JT, Rosenberg ZS. Entrapment neuropathies of the shoulder and elbow in the athlete. Clin Sports Med 2006;25(3):465–8.

11. Plancher KD, Luke TA, Peterson RK, et al. Posterior shoulder pain: a dynamic study of the spinoglenoid ligament and treatment with arthroscopic release of the scapular tunnel. Arthroscopy 2007;23:991–8.

12. Sanders TG, Tirman PF. Paralabral cyst: an unusual cause of quadrilateral space syndrome. Arthroscopy 1999;15:631–7.

13. Dumitru D, Zwarts MJ. Focal peripheral neuropathies. In: Dumitru D, Amato AA, Zwarts M, editors. Electrodiagnostic medicine. 2nd edition. Philadelphia: Hanley& Belfus, Inc; 2002. p. 225–56.

14. Dang AC, Rodner CM. Unusual compression neuropathies of the forearm, part I: radial nerve. J Hand Surg Am 2009;34(10):1906–14.

15. Submrony SH. Electrophysiological findings in crutch palsy. Electromyogr Clin Neurophysiol 1989; 29:281–5, tourniquet.

16. Bolton FB, McFarlane RM. Human pneumatic tourniquet paralysis. Neurology 1978;28:787–93.

17. Uchida Y, Sugioka Y. Ulnar nerve palsy after supracondylar humerus fracture. Acta Orthop Scand 1990;61:118–9.

18. Miller RG. The cubital tunnel syndrome: diagnosis and precise localization. Ann Neurol 1979;6:56–9.

19. Campbell WW, Carroll DJ, Greenbeg MK, et al. AAEM Quality Assurance Committee, et al. Practice parameter: electrodiagnostic studies in ulnar neuropathy at the elbow. Neurology 1999;52:688–90.

20. Spinner M. Injuries to the major branches of peripheral nerves of the forearm. Philadelphia: WB Saunders; 1978. p. 160–227.

21. Werner RA, Andary M. Electrodiagnostic evaluation of carpal tunnel syndrome. Muscle Nerve 2011; 44(4):597–607.

22. Hartz CR, Linscheid RL, Gramse RR, et al. The pronator teres syndrome: compressive neuropathy of the median nerve. J Bone Joint Surg Am 1981; 63(6):885–91.

23. Kimura J. Mononeuropathies and entrapment syndromes. In: Kimura, editor. Electrodiagnosis in diseases of nerve and muscle: principles and practice. 2nd edition. Philadelphia: FA Davis; 1989. p. 495–516.

24. Seitz WH Jr, Matsuoka H, McAdoo J, et al. Acute compression of the median nerve at the elbow by the lacertus fibrosus. J Shoulder Elbow Surg 2007; 16(1):91–4.

25. Nagano A. Spontaneous anterior interosseous nerve palsy. J Bone Joint Surg Br 2003;85(3):313–8.

Physical Examination of Upper Extremity Compressive Neuropathies

Samuel P. Popinchalk, MD, Alyssa A. Schaffer, MD*

KEYWORDS

- Compressive neuropathy • Physical examination • Radial neuropathy • Median neuropathy
- Ulnar neuropathy

KEY POINTS

- Upper extremity compressive neuropathies remain a clinical diagnosis, with scant high-level evidence to offer guidance.
- A thorough understanding of the anatomic course of the median, ulnar, and radial nerves are required to effectively perform a physical examination.
- Provocative maneuvers targeting the potential sites of compression are essential to locate the site of pathology.
- Electrodiagnostic testing is not without limitations, and therefore a thorough history and physical examination is essential to form the most accurate clinical picture.

INTRODUCTION

The primacy of anatomy cannot be understated with respect to the clinical diagnosis of compressive neuropathies. The examiner must assess motor and sensibility function of the nerve in question, as well as perform provocative maneuvers that may elicit neurologic symptoms. Evaluation should begin with a detailed history, as this is essential to formulate a differential diagnosis and guide physical examination.

Physical examination is fundamentally subjective; therefore, little evidence exists regarding the reliability and validity of physical examination for the upper extremity.[1] Electrodiagnostic studies represent the best source of objective data for the diagnosis of chronic nerve compression.[2,3] Electrodiagnostic testing is not without limitations, and therefore a thorough history and physical examination, with selected diagnostic testing, combine to form the most accurate clinical picture.

MEDIAN NERVE

Anatomy

The medial and lateral cords of the brachial plexus, which have contributions from the sixth, seventh, and eighth cervical and the first thoracic nerve roots form the median nerve. In the upper arm, the course of the median nerve is in close proximity to the brachial artery, both of which pass along the anterior aspect of the intermuscular septum on the medial side of the arm. The median nerve and brachial artery enter the antecubital fossa medial to the biceps brachii and superficial to the brachialis muscle, then course through three successive arches as they enter the forearm. Each of these arches represents a potential site of nerve compression.

Funding sources: None.
Conflict of interest: Dr Schaffer: Scientific Advisory Board of GenOssis LLC. Dr Popinchalk: None.
Department of Orthopaedic Surgery and Sports Medicine, Temple University, 3401 North Broad Street, Philadelphia, PA 19140, USA
* Corresponding author.
E-mail address: Alyssa.Schaffer@tuhs.temple.edu

Orthop Clin N Am 43 (2012) 417–430
http://dx.doi.org/10.1016/j.ocl.2012.07.011

The first arch is formed by the bicipital aponeurosis (lacertus fibrosis) as it connects the biceps brachii to the flexor-pronator mass and the ulna. The median nerve is superficial to the brachialis tendon, but deep to the bicipital aponeurosis. The two heads of the pronator teres (PT) muscle form the second arch. The median nerve lies superficial to the ulnar head and deep to the humeral head. Finally, the median nerve travels between the humeroulnar and radial heads of the flexor digitorum superficialis (FDS) muscle, under the thick fibrous structure between them, known as the sublimis ridge.

In the forearm, the median nerve runs along the radial side of the flexor digitorum profundus (FDP), deep to the FDS. The anterior interosseus nerve (AIN) branches from the median nerve in the proximal half of the forearm. True to its name, the anterior interosseus nerve runs along the anterior, or volar, aspect of the interosseous membrane before terminating deep to the pronator quadratus (PQ) muscle. At approximately five cm proximal to the wrist crease, the median nerve emerges superficially between the flexor carpi radialis (FCR) tendon radially and the palmaris longus (PL) tendon ulnarly. The PL is reportedly absent in approximately 5% to 65% of the population, with wide variation across ethnic lines.[4] The palmar cutaneous branch of the median nerve arises approximately five cm proximal to the distal wrist crease and passes outside of the carpal tunnel.

The median nerve then crosses the wrist as the most superficial of the 10 structures traversing the carpal tunnel. The transverse carpal ligament forms the roof of carpal tunnel volarly. The hook of the hamate, pisiform, and triquetrum form the ulnar wall, and the distal pole of the scaphoid and tubercle of the trapezium form the radial wall of the carpal tunnel.

Once in the hand, the thenar motor branch (or recurrent motor branch) emerges radially. The median nerve goes on to divide into radial and ulnar divisions in the plane between the flexor tendons (deep), and the palmar arch (superficially). The radial division splits to form the common digital nerve to the thumb and the proper digital nerve to the radial half of the index finger. The ulnar division splits to form the common digital nerves of the second and third web spaces.

Physical Examination

The median nerve innervates muscles involved in forearm pronation, wrist flexion, flexion of the digits, and thumb opposition and abduction (**Table 1**). The median nerve carries sensory innervation from the radial aspect of the palm via the palmar cutaneous branch, and the volar surfaces of the thumb, index,

middle fingers, and the radial half of the ring finger. Sensibility, therefore, is best tested over the thenar eminence to assess the palmar cutaneous branch and over the volar aspect of the distal index and middle fingers to assess the sensory fibers that pass through the carpal tunnel. This sensory information is essential for fine motor tasks.

Compressive Neuropathies of the Median Nerve

The ligament of Struthers
Approximately 1% of people have an accessory condyle or supracondylar spur approximately five cm proximal to the medial epicondyle of the humerus.[5] The ligament of Struthers attaches this bony prominence proximally to the medial epicondyle distally. The median nerve is susceptible to compression as it passes underneath this ligament along with the brachial artery. The patient will often complain of a deep aching pain in the proximal forearm with an insidious onset, hand weakness, and numbness in the median-nerve distribution. On examination, this pain is often exacerbated with testing of the PT and FCR. Worsening of symptoms often occurs with repetitive pronation and supination. The ability to palpate this bony prominence on physical examination is variable, depending on the patient's body habitus. Radiographs can reveal the supracondylar spur if palpation is equivocal. These patients can present with paresthesia or numbness in the median-nerve distribution as well as weakness in all muscles innervated by the median nerve, although frequently weakness of muscles innervated by the AIN is most prominent. A Tinel sign may be present proximal to the medial epicondyle. Compression of the median nerve as it passes under the bicipital aponeurosis is rare and may present similarly to compression at the ligament of Struthers.[6]

Pronator syndrome
Pronator syndrome results from compression of the median nerve as it passes between the 2 heads of the PT.[7] The patient often complains of aching discomfort in the forearm, weakness in the hand, and numbness in the thumb and index finger.[8] Commonly the patient will report a history of performing forceful repetitive forearm pronation movements. On physical examination, tenderness on palpation of the PT muscle is a common finding. A Tinel sign may be present in the antecubital fossa. Testing of motor function can be difficult secondary to pain. The PT muscle receives its innervation proximal to the site of compression, and therefore might be the only muscle innervated by the median nerve spared in this syndrome. The Phalen test may be positive in 50% of patients with

Table 1
Median nerve: motor innervation

Muscle	Innervation	Action	Examination
Pronator teres	Median nerve	Forearm pronation (primary)	Resisted forearm supination, with the forearm fully pronated and the elbow extended
Flexor carpi radialis	Median nerve	Wrist flexion, radial deviation	Palpation of FCR with resisted wrist flexion with palpation of muscle belly
Palmaris longus	Median nerve	Wrist flexion (weak)	Palpation of PL tendon with resisted wrist flexion
Flexor digitorum Superficialis	Median nerve	PIP joint flexion	Resisted PIP joint flexion (sequential) while remaining fingers in extension, and the wrist at neutral
Flexor digitorum profundus (index & middle)	AIN	DIP joint flexion of the index, long, ring, and small fingers	Index DIP joint flexion while the MCP and PIP joints are held in extension
Flexor pollicis longus	AIN	Thumb IP joint flexion	Thumb IP joint flexion with MCP joint stabilized
Pronator quadratus	AIN	Forearm pronation (secondary)	Resisted forearm pronation with elbow flexed to isolate PQ from the PT
Abductor pollicis brevis	Median nerve	Palmar thumb abduction	Resisted abduction in the plane perpendicular to the palm with the remaining metacarpals stabilized
Flexor pollicis brevis (superficial head)	Median nerve	Thumb MCP joint flexion	Flexion of thumb MCP joint with IP joint held in extension to isolate from FPL
Opponens pollicis	Median nerve	Thumb opposition	Opposition of the volar pads of the thumb and small finger, while the examiner attempts pull the thumb away
Lumbricals (first and second)	Median nerve	MCP joint flexion, PIP and DIP joint extension (index and long)	Resisted extension of the PIP joint with MCP joint hyperextended (cannot isolate from interosseous muscles)

Abbreviations: AIN, anterior interosseus nerve; DIP, distal interphalangeal; FCR, flexor carpi radialis; FPL, flexor pollicis longus; IP, interphalangeal; MCP, metacarpophalangeal; PIP, proximal interphalangeal; PL, palmaris longus; PQ, pronator quadratus; PT, pronator teres.

pronator syndrome, and therefore is unreliable in distinguishing pronator syndrome from carpal tunnel syndrome (CTS).[8] Unlike CTS, a history of nocturnal pain and/or numbness is rare. Another provocative maneuver to test for in pronator syndrome is to apply direct pressure in the area of the PT with the patient's forearm supinated. It is considered positive if paresthesia is reported in the median nerve distribution within one minute of compression (**Fig. 1**).

The next possible site of compression along the course of the median nerve is the sublimis arch

formed between the two heads of the FDS. Again, clinical findings are similar to those in pronator syndrome, although pain exacerbated by strong flexion of the proximal interphalangeal joints of the index, long, ring, and little fingers is suggestive of compression at the sublimis arch rather than at the PT.[9]

Anterior interosseous nerve syndrome
AIN syndrome is an uncommon disease of unknown etiology and pathophysiology.[10] Patients may describe vague proximal forearm pain and

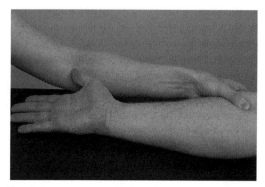

Fig. 1. Pronator compression test. Direct pressure on the proximal forearm over the pronator teres muscle reproduces or exacerbates paresthesia or numbness in the distribution of the median nerve.

progressive loss in their ability to do tasks requiring fine motor control and pinch, such as handwriting. On physical examination, the patient will have weakness in the FDP to the index and middle fingers and weakness in the PQ. Deficits in the flexor pollicis longus (FPL) and index-finger FDP result in the inability to form the "OK" sign. The patient will only be able to contact the volar pads of their thumb and index fingers, rather than the tips, without flexion of the thumb interphalangeal and index distal interphalangeal joints. Sensibility is normal, as the AIN does not contain sensory fibers to the hand. Symptoms of AIN syndrome can be provoked with resisted elbow flexion, resisted forearm pronation, and resisted finger flexion (**Fig. 2**).

Carpal tunnel syndrome

CTS results from compression of the median nerve as it travels beneath the transverse carpal ligament. The prevalence of CTS in the general population of the United States is estimated at 3.72%.[11]

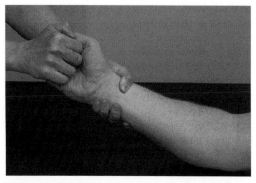

Fig. 2. Provocative maneuver for anterior interosseus nerve syndrome. Resisted elbow flexion, forearm pronation, and finger flexion elicits temporary weakness of finger flexion.

CTS remains a clinical diagnosis; as there exists no gold standard test for its diagnosis. The lack of clear diagnostic standards contributes to the fact that treatment failure for CTS most commonly results from erroneous diagnosis.[12,13]

Physical examination is a critical source of information in the diagnosis of CTS, although its utility as a screening tool has been questioned.[14] Therefore, historical findings consistent with CTS are fundamental to its clinical diagnosis. Patients predominantly complain of numbness and/or paresthesia in the median-nerve distribution, rather than pain. These symptoms are typically worse at night and are improved with shaking of the hand, known as the flick sign. Patients may describe discomfort in the thenar eminence. A history of dropping objects correlates with weakness of the opponens pollicis and abductor pollicis brevis muscles. Atrophy of these thenar muscles represents advanced disease. Selected physical examination findings for the evaluation of CTS are described in **Table 2**.

The American Academy of Orthopaedic Surgeons (AAOS) published recommendations for diagnosing CTS based on a comprehensive review of the literature. With respect to physical examination, the level of evidence was poor because the studies are predominantly of a case-control variety, and significant variation existed in the testing maneuver protocols.[15] The highest-level recommendation made by the AAOS group is to obtain electrodiagnostic testing if clinical evaluation is positive and surgical management is being considered. This recommendation remains controversial, as some investigators claim electrodiagnostic tests do not change the probability of diagnosing CTS in patients who are considered to have CTS based on their history and physical examination alone.[16] In 2006, Graham[2] used a panel of experts to assess the diagnostic utility of 57 clinical findings associated with CTS. Two historical and 4 physical examination findings had a statistically significant correlation with expert consensus diagnosis of CTS, and are referred to as the CTS-6 (**Box 1**).

ULNAR NERVE
Anatomy

The Ulnar nerve is a continuation of the medial cord of the brachial plexus, which has contributions from the eighth cervical and first thoracic nerve roots. The ulnar nerve travels on the anterior border of the intermuscular septum, medial to the brachial artery, which is medial to the median nerve. At the midpoint of the humerus, the nerve pierces the intermuscular septum, entering the medial head of the triceps brachii. In 70% of people, the nerve then passes under the arcade of Struthers.[36] The

Table 2
Physical examination findings of CTS

Test	Procedure	Positive Result	Sensitivity/ Specificity
Phalen wrist flexion test[17,18]	Maximal flexion of wrists by opposing dorsal surfaces of hands (**Fig. 3**)	Reproduction or exacerbation of paresthesia or numbness in median nerve distribution within 60 s	(0.46–0.80)/ (0.51–0.91)[19–22]
Durkin carpal compression test[23]	Exert direct pressure at or just proximal to the carpal tunnel (**Fig. 4**)	Reproduction or exacerbation of paresthesia or numbness in the median nerve distribution within 60 s	(0.04–0.79)/ (0.25–0.96)[19,22,24]
Tinel sign[25,26]	Light tapping over the median nerve at the wrist	Reproduction or exacerbation of paresthesia in the median nerve distribution	(0.28–0.73)/ (0.44–0.95)[19–21,27]
Static 2-point discrimination testing[28]	Two points of various distance are applied with just enough pressure for patient to appreciate the stimulus	Inability to distinguish 2 points 5 mm apart	(0.06–0.28)/ (0.98)[29–31,a]
Semmes-Weinstein monofilament testing[32,33]	Monofilaments of varying diameters are applied to volar aspect of distal index or middle finger until the filament bends	Inability to perceive a monofilament sized 2.83 or less	(0.59–0.83)/ (0.59)[30,31,34,a]
Ten test[35]	A score (1–10) is reported by the patient comparing an area of abnormal light touch sensibility in the median nerve distribution to an area of similar innervation density with intact light touch sensibility	Ratio less than one between abnormal (scored 1–9) vs normal area (scored 10). Allows examiner to track changes over time	No data available

[a] Only one specificity value reported.

Box 1
CTS-6 clinical findings

1. Numbness/paresthesia predominantly in median-nerve territory
2. Nocturnal numbness
3. Thenar atrophy and/or weakness
4. Positive Phalen test
5. Loss of 2-point discrimination
6. Positive Tinel sign

Data from Graham B, Regehr G, Naglie G, et al. Development and validation of diagnostic criteria for carpal tunnel syndrome. J Hand Surg Am 2006;31:919–24.

arcade of Struthers is an aponeurotic band connecting the intramuscular septum to the medial head of the triceps, and is located approximately eight cm proximal to the medial epicondyle of the humerus. The ulnar nerve then becomes superficial as it crosses the posteromedial aspect of the elbow joint in the postcondylar groove. The medial epicondyle of the humerus (anterior and medial), the olecranon process of the ulna (posterior and lateral), and the ulnohumeral ligament (lateral) form this fibro-osseous canal.

The ulnar nerve enters the forearm between the humeral and ulnar heads of the flexor carpi ulnaris (FCU). This passageway is known as the cubital tunnel, made up of the Osborne ligament (the aponeurosis between the 2 heads of the FCU)

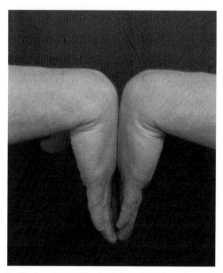

Fig. 3. Phalen (wrist flexion) test. Holding the wrists in maximal flexion for up to 60 seconds reproduces or exacerbates paresthesia or numbness in the median nerve distribution in the hand. The method demonstrated is a modification of Phalen's originally described procedure, which used gravity alone to flex the wrist.

and then the 2 heads of the FCU. After innervating and traversing the FCU, the ulnar nerve runs superficial to FDP, innervating the FDP muscles to the ring and little fingers. The ulnar nerve courses between the FCU and FDP tendons, becoming superficial in the distal forearm.

The ulnar nerve enters the hand via the Guyon canal, passing between the transverse carpal ligament deep and the volar carpal ligament superficially, before its bifurcation into the superficial sensory and deep motor divisions. The deep motor division courses deep to the origin of the hypothenar musculature on the hook of the hamate, innervating the hypothenar muscles, the

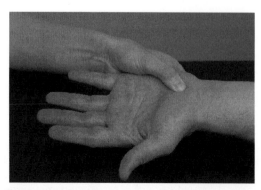

Fig. 4. Carpal compression test. Exert direct pressure at or just proximal to the carpal tunnel. A positive test will reproduce or exacerbate paresthesia or numbness in the median nerve distribution.

interossei, the third and fourth lumbricals, and the adductor pollicis brevis and flexor pollicis brevis. The superficial sensory branch runs along the volar surface of the hypothenar muscles, innervating the palmaris brevis, the ulnar half of the ring finger, and the little finger.

Physical Examination

The ulnar nerve innervates muscles involved in wrist and finger flexion, as well as most of the hand intrinsic muscles (**Table 3**). The ulnar nerve receives information from three sensory branches covering the ulnar third of the hand. The dorsal ulnar cutaneous nerve emerges deep to the FCU tendon approximately 5 to 10 cm proximal to the wrist crease, innervating the dorso-ulnar hand and the dorsum of the little finger and the ulnar half of the ring finger proximal to the distal interphalangeal (DIP) joints. The superficial sensory division innervates the volar aspect of the ring and ulnar half of the little finger and the more distal dorsal aspect of those fingers, distal to the DIP joints. Next, the palmar ulnar cutaneous branch of the ulnar nerve innervates the ulnar one-third of the palm. Assessing the skin over the hypothenar eminence best tests the palmar ulnar cutaneous branch.

Compressive Neuropathies of the Ulnar Nerve

Ulnar-nerve entrapment is the second most common compressive neuropathy of the upper extremity.[37] The most common sites of compression of the ulnar nerve are the cubital tunnel at the elbow and the Guyon canal at the wrist. With knowledge of the course of the ulnar nerve, the pattern of sensory and motor findings is crucial not only to diagnosis but also to differentiating between common sites of compression. For example, if sensibility in the dorsal ulnar cutaneous distribution is spared, but sensibility in the distribution of the superficial sensory division of the ulnar nerve is compromised, compression within the Guyon canal is suspected.

McGowan[38] proposed a classification system for ulnar neuropathies that can be applied without regard to the level at which the nerve is compressed. This classification system is graded in terms of motor involvement. Grade I lesions are associated with paresthesia and numbness but no weakness. Grade II lesions are associated with weakness and early atrophy of the interosseous musculature. Grade III lesions represent a more advanced level of weakness with complete paralysis of hand intrinsic muscles.

Characteristic physical examination signs indicating ulnar-nerve dysfunction include the inability

Table 3
Ulnar nerve: motor innervation

Muscle	Innervation	Action	Examination
Flexor carpi ulnaris	Ulnar nerve	Wrist flexion and ulnar deviation	Resisted ulnar wrist flexion or palpation of FCU tendon with little finger abduction. The FCU functions to stabilize the pisiform to provide a stable base from which the abductor digiti minimi can work
Flexor digitorum profundus	Ulnar nerve	DIP joint flexion of the ring, and small fingers	Ring DIP joint flexion while the MCP and PIP joints are held in extension
Palmaris brevis	Superficial sensory division of ulnar nerve	Tenses hypothenar skin	Skin corrugation over hypothenar eminence with little finger abduction
Abductor digiti minimi	Deep motor division of ulnar nerve	Little finger abduction	Gently resisted little finger abduction
Flexor digiti minimi	Deep motor division of ulnar nerve	Little finger MCP joint flexion	Flexion of the little finger MCP joint with the interphalangeal joints extended (cannot be isolated from lumbrical and palmar interosseous to little finger)
Opponens digiti minimi	Deep motor division of Ulnar nerve	Small finger MCP joint flexion and supination	Opposition of the volar pads of the thumb and small finger, while the examiner attempts pull the little finger away
Lumbricals (third & fourth)	Deep motor division of ulnar nerve	MCP joint flexion, PIP and DIP joint extension (ring and little)	Resisted extension of the PIP joint with MCP joint hyperextended (cannot isolate from interosseous muscles)
Palmar interossei	Deep motor division of ulnar nerve	Finger adduction and MCP joint flexion, PIP and DIP joint extension	Finger adduction against resistance
Dorsal interossei	Deep motor division of ulnar nerve	Finger abduction	Finger abduction against resistance
Adductor pollicis	Deep motor division of ulnar nerve	Thumb adduction	Maintain thumb adduction against radial palm against resistance with IP joint extended
Flexor pollicis brevis (deep head)	Deep motor division of ulnar nerve	Thumb MCP joint flexion	Flexion of thumb MCP joint with IP joint held in extension to isolate from FPL

Abbreviation: FCU, flexor carpi ulnaris.

to cross the index and middle fingers, Duchenne sign, Wartenberg sign, and Froment sign. The Duchenne sign is clawing of the ring and little finger when the patient is asked to open the hand. The loss of function of the flexor digiti minimi, as well as the lumbrical and interossei muscles to the ring and little finger, results in clawing, or relative extension of the metacarpophalangeal (MCP) joints, and flexion of the interphalangeal joints. The Wartenberg sign is relative abduction of the little finger when the patient is asked to extend the fingers. Without the function of the third palmar interosseous muscle to adduct the little finger, the extensor digiti minimi (EDM) and extensor digitorum communis (EDC) slightly abduct the little finger as it extends. When asked to adduct the little finger to the ring finger, the patient will be unable to do so. The Froment sign is demonstrated by the inability to clasp a piece of paper between the thumb and the radial aspect of the index finger with the thumb interphalangeal joint extended. A positive Froment sign is produced by substitution of the FPL for the adductor pollicis, resulting in flexion of the interphalangeal joint. More advanced disease will result in atrophy of the intrinsic muscles. This atrophy is best demonstrated by comparing the first dorsal interosseous or hypothenar muscle mass with the unaffected side.

Cubital tunnel syndrome

The ulnar nerve is at its most vulnerable as it traverses the elbow joint, making ulnar nerve compression at the cubital tunnel the second most prevalent upper extremity compression neuropathy.[39] Compression can occur for a variety of reasons and at several points about the elbow, from the arcade of Struthers to the Osbourne ligament. The volume of this channel is decreased with elbow flexion; therefore, irritation at this site is associated with repetitive tasks requiring elbow flexion. This reduction in volume with elbow flexion results in an increase in pressure within the cubital tunnel, possibly leading to relative ischemia of the ulnar nerve.[40] Cubital tunnel syndrome is also associated with recurrent subluxation of the ulnar nerve with deep elbow flexion. This hypermobility of the ulnar nerve is usually bilateral and is present in up to 20% of the population.[41]

The diagnosis of cubital tunnel syndrome is primarily clinical. Patients will complain of paresthesia in the small and ring finger. Motor deficits are consistent with more advanced disease. Evaluation begins with inspection of the elbow looking for deformity, carrying angle, and range of motion. While assessing flexion and extension of the elbow, the ulnar nerve should be palpated to rule out subluxation. After assessing motor and sensibility function, provocative testing (cubital tunnel compression test, Tinel sign, and the scratch collapse test) can help delineate the level of the ulnar nerve lesion, as well as severity.

In early disease, the provocative tests may be the only positive clinical findings.[42] The Tinel sign is often positive at the level of the cubital tunnel, but this test is not as specific as the cubital tunnel compression test. This test is performed by assisting maximal flexion of the elbow while applying direct pressure on the ulnar nerve just proximal to the cubital tunnel. As with all provocative maneuvers, the test is positive if

paresthesia is induced or exacerbated within 1 minute of pressure being applied (**Fig. 5**). This test is reportedly positive in up to 10% of normal individuals.[43] The scratch collapse test is performed with the arm adducted and the elbow flexed. The patient externally rotates the shoulder against resistance while the examiner gently scratches the skin overlying the cubital tunnel. A positive result is demonstrated when momentary loss of external rotation strength occurs after the skin overlying the site of compression is stimulated.[44] The scratch collapse test is reported to be significantly more sensitive than the Tinel sign and cubital tunnel compression testing for cubital tunnel syndrome.[21]

Guyon canal (ulnar tunnel) syndrome

Guyon described the course of the ulnar nerve as it crossed the wrist joint in 1861, identifying it as a potential site for compression.[45] Compression in the Guyon canal is divided into three zones. Compression in zone 1 results in mixed motor and sensory disturbances, as this zone is proximal to the bifurcation of the ulnar nerve. Compression in zone 2 involves the deep motor branch of the ulnar nerve, and therefore motor function distal to the Guyon canal will be compromised while the superficial sensory branch remains unaffected; this is the most common site of compression. Compression in zone 3 of the canal results in

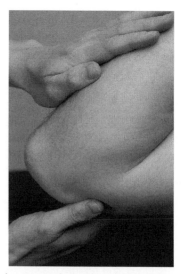

Fig. 5. Ulnar nerve (cubital tunnel) compression test. Direct pressure over the cubital tunnel with elbow maximally flexed reproduces or exacerbates paresthesia or numbness in the ulnar nerve distribution. Palpation of the ulnar nerve is required to ensure the nerve has not subluxed from its normal course through the cubital tunnel.

isolated sensory changes caused by compression of the superficial sensory branch only.[46]

Compression within the Guyon canal, as opposed to the cubital tunnel, should be suspected when sensibility is spared in the distribution of the dorsal ulnar cutaneous branch of the ulnar nerve. This nerve crosses the wrist outside the Guyon canal and, depending on the etiology of compression, may be spared. Paresthesia or numbness can be provoked with direct pressure over the Guyon canal at the wrist (**Fig. 6**).

RADIAL NERVE
Anatomy

The radial nerve is the continuance of the posterior cord of the brachial plexus, communicating with the fifth, sixth, seventh, and eighth cervical nerve roots, and is the largest of the terminal branches of the brachial plexus. Initially the radial nerve travels posterior to the axillary artery and along the anterior aspect of the long head of the triceps. The radial nerve reaches the spiral groove of the humerus by descending laterally and posteriorly between the long (superficial) and medial (deep) heads of the triceps, where it runs between their origins. The long head of the triceps is believed to be the first muscle innervated by the radial nerve, although de Seze and colleagues,[47] in an anatomic and electromyographic study, found this motor branch to arise from the axillary nerve near its origin. The motor branches to the lateral and medial heads of the triceps brachii arise from the radial nerve before it enters the spiral groove. The radial nerve then reaches the anterior compartment of the arm by penetrating the lateral intermuscular septum just distal to the deltoid insertion at the midpoint of the humerus. At this point, the radial nerve enters the radial tunnel.

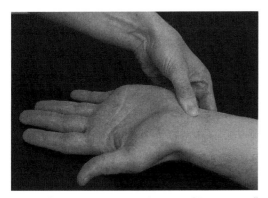

Fig. 6. Ulnar nerve compression test (Guyon canal). Direct pressure proximal to Guyon canal reproduces or exacerbates paresthesia or numbness in the ulnar nerve distribution.

The radial tunnel is formed laterally by the muscles of the mobile wad (the brachioradialis [BR], the extensor carpi radialis longus [ECRL], and the extensor carpi radialis brevis [ECRB]), medially by the biceps tendon and brachialis, and posteriorly by the radiocapitellar joint capsule.[48] The BR muscle proximally lies lateral to the radial nerve but, as the muscle proceeds distally, passes anteriorly over the nerve to form the roof of the tunnel. The radial nerve remains anterior to the lateral epicondyle of the humerus and anterior and lateral to the brachialis tendon as it enters the forearm. The motor branches to the BR and ECRL muscles arise proximal to the lateral epicondyle of the humerus while the motor branch to the ECRB arises distal to the lateral epicondyle. The superficial sensory branch arises from the main radial nerve before it continues as the posterior interosseous nerve (PIN). Most commonly, this bifurcation occurs in the proximal forearm just before the PIN passes under the arcade of Frohse. The arcade of Frohse, also known as the supinator arch, is the tendinous connection between the deep and superficial heads of the supinator muscle.[49] The motor branch to the supinator muscle arises from the PIN before passage under the arcade of Frohse. Subsequent to its passage through the arcade of Frohse, the PIN innervates the extensor carpi ulnaris muscle. The PIN continues through the supinator muscle as it travels from the anterior to the dorsal compartment of the forearm.

After exiting the supinator muscle, the PIN divides into a deep branch, which innervates the abductor pollicis longus, extensor pollicis longus (EPL), extensor pollicis brevis (EPB), and extensor indicis proprius (EIP) muscles, and a superficial branch, which innervates the extensor carpi ulnaris (ECU), extensor digitorum communis (EDC), and extensor digiti quinti (EDQ) muscles. The superficial sensory radial nerve courses deep to the BR muscle, and emerges between the ECRL and BR tendons.

Physical Examination

The radial nerve innervates the extensor muscles in the arm and forearm. The radial nerve innervates the triceps brachii and the three muscles of the mobile wad and, via the PIN, the seven muscles in the dorsal compartments of the forearm (**Table 4**).

The first sensory branch of the radial nerve is the posterior cutaneous nerve to the arm. Loss of sensibility in this territory (posterior arm) is consistent with a radial nerve injury proximal to the spiral groove of the humerus.

Table 4
Radial nerve: motor innervation

Muscle	Innervation	Action	Examination
Triceps brachii	Radial nerve	Elbow extension	Resisted elbow extension
Brachioradialis	Radial nerve	Elbow flexion with forearm in neutral, and brings forearm into neutral from either pronation or supination	Resisted elbow flexion with the forearm in neutral rotation while palpating the muscle belly
Extensor carpi radialis longus	Radial nerve	Wrist extension and radial deviation	Resisted wrist extension and radial deviation with forearm stabilized in pronation
Extensor carpi radialis brevis	Radial nerve	Wrist extension and radial deviation	Resisted wrist extension and radial deviation with forearm stabilized in pronation
Supinator	PIN	Forearm supination	Resisted forearm supination
Extensor carpi ulnaris	PIN	Wrist extension and ulnar deviation	Wrist extension and ulnar deviation against resistance with DIP and PIP joints relaxed
Extensor digitorum communis	PIN	MCP joint extension (index, middle, ring, little)	Resisted extension of these 4 joints in sequence (the wrist must not flex during this assessment, as passive extension of the MCP occurs due to tenodesis effect)
Extensor digiti minimi	PIN	Little finger MCP joint extension (accessory)	Same as EDC to little finger (normally weak, compare with contralateral side)
Abductor pollicis longus	PIN	Thumb carpometacarpal joint abduction in plane of the palm	Resisted thumb abduction in plane of palm with thumb IP and MCP joints already in extension to isolate from EPL and EPB
Extensor pollicis longus	PIN	Thumb IP joint extension	Resisted thumb IP joint extension
Extensor pollicis brevis	PIN	Thumb MCP joint extension	Resisted thumb MCP joint extension with IP joint relaxed
Extensor indicis	PIN	Index MCP joint extension (accessory)	Same as EDC to index (cannot be isolated)

Abbreviations: EDC, extensor digitorum communis; EPB, extensor pollicis brevis; EPL, extensor pollicis longus; PIN, posterior interosseous nerve.

The lower lateral cutaneous nerve to the arm innervates the lateral arm distal to the deltoid. If sensibility in this region is impaired, but sensibility in the distribution of the posterior cutaneous nerve to the arm is intact, radial nerve injury in the spiral groove of the humerus is suspected.

The posterior cutaneous nerve to the forearm receives sensory information from the dorsolateral aspect of the forearm. This nerve courses with the radial nerve in the spiral groove of the humerus, pierces the brachial fascia at the lateral intermuscular septum, and passes posteriorly to the lateral epicondyle.

The territory of the superficial sensory radial nerve is the dorsoradial half of the hand, including the index, middle, and radial half of the ring finger proximal to their DIP joints and the dorsum of the thumb proximal to the interphalangeal joint. This nerve is best assessed in the first dorsal web space between the thumb and index fingers.

Compressive Neuropathies of the Radial Nerve

Extension of the elbow, wrist, and fingers is requisite to placing the hand in a functionally useful position; therefore, radial nerve dysfunction can be debilitating. More distal compression syndromes can be easily distinguished from posterior cord abnormality based on the presence of deltoid and latissimus dorsi muscle function. These muscles are innervated by the axillary nerve and thoracodorsal nerves, respectively, both of which branch from the posterior cord of the brachial plexus.

Posterior interosseous nerve syndrome

PIN compression can occur at multiple points, the arcade of Frohse being the most common.[50–55] The clinical presentation of PIN syndrome is related to motor complaints, as the PIN is primarily a motor nerve. Barring a history of trauma, patients will often complain of a dull aching pain in the muscle belly of the supinator.[56] Innervation to the supinator muscle is often spared, but innervation of ECU, EDC, EDM, abductor pollicis longus, EPL, EPB, and extensor indicis will be compromised. On examination, patients will lack strength (partially or completely) with thumb extension and extension of the MCP joints.[57] Also, because ECRL and ECRB innervation will not be affected, radial deviation of the wrist will be observed with wrist extension.[58,59] Provocative maneuvers include the supinator compression and resisted middle finger extension tests (**Figs. 7** and **8**).

Radial tunnel syndrome

Radial tunnel syndrome is somewhat of a controversial diagnosis. Rosenbaum stated:

> There is no debate that some cases of posterior interosseous nerve (PIN) palsy, manifest by definite weakness in muscles innervated by the PIN, are caused by nerve entrapment in the radial tunnel; the arguable issue is

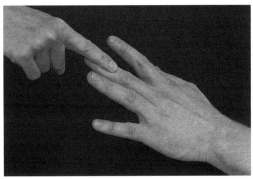

Fig. 8. Resisted middle finger and wrist extension test. The examiner resists middle finger and wrist extension, thereby reproducing pain in the proximal forearm or exacerbating weakness of these PIN-innervated actions.

> whether there is a distinctive radial tunnel syndrome of forearm pain and tenderness, unassociated with muscle weakness, that is caused by nerve entrapment in the radial tunnel.[60]

Rosenbaum described "disputed radial tunnel syndrome" as a condition characterized by complaints of pain over the lateral aspect of the forearm, especially after activities requiring forceful elbow extension or forearm rotation. The patient may complain of weakness after activities, which is thought to be secondary to pain, and not true weakness.[45] The true etiology is debated, but thought to be secondary to entrapment of the PIN in the radial tunnel. Radial tunnel syndrome can be distinguished from PIN syndrome based on the absence of true weakness. Furthermore, lateral epicondylitis must be ruled out as a possible cause.

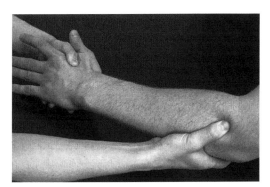

Fig. 7. Supinator compression test at the arcade of Frohse. Direct pressure on the proximal forearm over the supinator muscle during resisted supination elicits temporary weakness of forearm supination or tenderness.

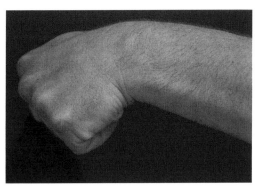

Fig. 9. Forearm pronation with wrist flexion and ulnar deviation reproduces or exacerbates paresthesia or numbness in the distribution of the SRN. This maneuver compresses the brachioradialis and extensor carpi radialis longus tendons between which the SRN emerges.

Radial tunnel syndrome is diagnosed by clinical findings of tenderness to palpation over the radial tunnel, pain with resisted extension of the middle finger, and pain with resisted forearm supination in the absence of muscle weakness. It is critical to compare findings to the contralateral asymptomatic arm and to test an area more proximal on the radial nerve to determine whether this also elicits tenderness to palpation. If these sites elicit a similar amount of tenderness to palpation, then a diagnosis of radial tunnel syndrome is less likely. Another useful diagnostic test is to block the PIN at the supinator with lidocaine to see whether the patient's pain is relieved. At another office visit, the lateral epicondyle can be injected to help distinguish between the two diagnoses.

Wartenberg (superficial radial nerve) compression

Superficial radial nerve (SRN) compression became known as Wartenberg syndrome after his publication of a case series of five patients with isolated neuropathy of the SRN.[61] Patients often complain of pain, numbness, or paresthesia in the radial sensory nerve distribution. These symptoms are exacerbated by forearm pronation and ulnar wrist flexion. Physical examination findings include a positive Tinel sign over the distal radial border of the forearm, and abnormal perception of light touch and abnormal two-point discrimination in the distribution of the SRN. A provocative maneuver mimicking the exacerbating activities should be performed after the sensibility examination. The patient is instructed to pronate the forearm and maximally flex and ulnarly deviate the wrist (**Fig. 9**).[62] This maneuver will entrap the SRN where it emerges between the brachioradialis

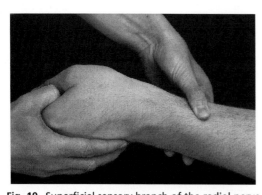

Fig. 10. Superficial sensory branch of the radial nerve compression test. Direct pressure at the junction of the brachioradialis and extensor carpi radialis longus tendons reproduces or exacerbates paresthesia or numbness in the distribution of the superficial sensory branch of the radial nerve.

and ECRL tendons. The superficial sensory branch of the radial nerve compression test is another provocative maneuver to evaluate for SRN compression, and is illustrated in **Fig. 10**.

SUMMARY

Upper extremity compressive neuropathies remain a clinical diagnosis, with scant high-level evidence to offer guidance. A thorough understanding of the anatomic course of the median, ulnar, and radial nerves as well as the provocative maneuvers targeting the potential sites of compression are required to effectively perform a physical examination, and ultimately to make the correct diagnosis.

REFERENCES

1. Marx RG, Bombardier C, Wright JG. What do we know about the reliability and validity of physical examination tests used to examine the upper extremity? J Hand Surg Am 1999;24:185–93.
2. Graham B. The value added by electrodiagnostic testing in the diagnosis of carpal tunnel syndrome. J Bone Joint Surg Am 2008;90:2587–93.
3. Strandberg EJ, Mozaffar T, Gupta R. The role of neurodiagnostic studies in nerve injuries and other orthopedic disorders. J Hand Surg Am 2007;32:1280–90.
4. Sebastin SJ, Lim AY, Bee WH, et al. Does the absence of the palmaris longus affect grip and pinch strength? J Hand Surg Br 2005;30(4):406–8.
5. Terry RJ. A study of the supracondyloid process in the living. Am J Phys Anthropol 1921;4:129–39.
6. Laha RK, Lunsford LD, Dujobny M. Lacertus fibrosus compression of the median nerve. J Neurosurg 1978;48:838–41.
7. Seyffarth H. Primary myoses in the m. pronator teres as cause of lesion of the n. medianus (the pronator syndrome). Acta Psychiatr Neurol Scand Suppl 1951;74:251–4.
8. Hartz C, Linscheid R. The pronator teres syndrome: compressive neuropathy of the median nerve. J Bone Joint Surg Am 1981;63:885–90.
9. Eversmann WW. Proximal median nerve compression. Hand Clin 1992;8:307–15.
10. Chi Y, Harness NG. Anterior interosseous nerve syndrome. J Hand Surg Am 2010;35(12):2078–80.
11. Papanicolaou GD, McCabe SJ, Firrell J. The prevalence and characteristics of nerve compression symptoms in the general population. J Hand Surg Am 2001;26:460–6.
12. Hunt TR, Osterman AL. Complications of the treatment of carpal tunnel syndrome. Hand Clin 1994;10:63–71.
13. Kessler FB. Complications of the management of carpal tunnel syndrome. Hand Clin 1986;2:401–6.

14. Dale AM, Descatha A, Coomes J, et al. Physical examination has a low yield in screening for carpal tunnel syndrome. Am J Ind Med 2011;54(1):1–9.

15. Keith MW, Masear V, Chung K, et al. Diagnosis of carpal tunnel syndrome. J Am Acad Orthop Surg 2009;17:389–96.

16. Graham B, Regehr G, Naglie G, et al. Development and validation of diagnostic criteria for carpal tunnel syndrome. J Hand Surg Am 2006;31:919–24.

17. Phalen GS. The carpal-tunnel syndrome. Seventeen years' experience in diagnosis and treatment of six hundred fifty-four hands. J Bone Joint Surg Am 1966;48:211–28.

18. Phalen GS. The carpal-tunnel syndrome. Clinical evaluation of 598 hands. Clin Orthop 1972;83:29–40.

19. de Krom MC, Knipschild PG, Kester AD, et al. Efficacy of provocative tests for diagnosis of carpal tunnel syndrome. Lancet 1990;335:393–5.

20. Raudino F. Tethered median nerve stress test in the diagnosis of carpal tunnel syndrome. Electromyogr Clin Neurophysiol 2000;40:57–60.

21. Katz JN, Larson MG, Sabra A, et al. The carpal tunnel syndrome: diagnostic utility of the history and physical examination findings. Ann Intern Med 1990;112:321–7.

22. Fertl E, Wober C, Zeitlhofer J. The serial use of two provocative tests in the clinical diagnosis of carpal tunnel syndrome. Acta Neurol Scand 1998;98: 328–32.

23. Durkan JA. A new diagnostic test for carpal tunnel syndrome. J Bone Joint Surg Am 1991;73(4):535–8.

24. Kaul MP, Pagel KJ, Wheatley MJ, et al. Carpal compression test and pressure provocative test in veterans with median-distribution paresthesias. Muscle Nerve 2001;24:107–11.

25. Tinel J. Le signe du "fourmillement"dans les lesions des nerfs peripheriques. Presse Med 1915;23: 388–9.

26. Stewart JD, Eisen A. Tinel's sign and the carpal tunnel syndrome. Br Med J 1978;2:1125–6.

27. Gomes I, Becker J, Ehlers JA, et al. Prediction of the neurophysiological diagnosis of carpal tunnel syndrome from the demographic and clinical data. Clin Neurophysiol 2006;117:964–71.

28. Moberg E. Objective methods for determining the functional value of sensibility in the hand. J Bone Joint Surg Br 1958;40(3):454–76.

29. Gerr F, Letz R. The sensitivity and specificity of tests for carpal tunnel syndrome vary with the comparison subjects. J Hand Surg Br 1998;23:151–5.

30. Buch-Jaeger N, Foucher G. Correlation of clinical signs with nerve conduction tests in the diagnosis of carpal tunnel syndrome. J Hand Surg Br 1994; 19:720–4.

31. Szabo RM, Gelberman RH, Dimick MP. Sensibility testing in patients with carpal tunnel syndrome. J Bone Joint Surg Am 1984;66:60–4.

32. Weinstein S. Tactile sensitivity of the phalanges. Percept Mot Skills 1962;14:351–4.

33. Levin S, Pearsall G, Ruderman RJ. Von Frey's method of measuring pressure sensibility in the hand: an engineering analysis of the Weinstein-Semmes pressure aesthesiometer. J Hand Surg Am 1978;3:211–6.

34. Spindler HA, Dellon AL. Nerve conduction studies and sensibility testing in carpal tunnel syndrome. J Hand Surg 1982;7:260–3.

35. Strauch B, Lang A, Ferder M, et al. The ten test. Plast Reconstr Surg 1997;99:1074.

36. Spinner M, Kaplan EB. The relationship of the ulnar nerve to the medial intermuscular septum in the arm and its clinical significance. Hand 1976;8(3): 239–42.

37. Elhassan B, Steinmann S. Entrapment neuropathy of the ulnar nerve. J Am Acad Orthop Surg 2007;15: 672–81.

38. McGowan AJ. The results of transposition of the ulnar nerve for traumatic ulnar neuritis. J Bone Joint Surg Br 1950;32:293–301.

39. Posner MA. Compressive ulnar neuropathies at the elbow: I. Etiology and diagnosis. J Am Acad Orthop Surg 1998;6:282–8.

40. Gelberman RH, Yamaguchi K, Hollstien SB, et al. Changes in interstitial pressure and cross-sectional area of the cubital tunnel and of the ulnar nerve with flexion of the elbow. J Bone Joint Surg Am 1998;80:492–501.

41. Childress HM. Recurrent ulnar-nerve dislocation at the elbow. Clin Orthop Relat Res 1975;108:168–73.

42. Novak CB, Lee GW, Mackinnon SE, et al. Provocative testing for cubital tunnel syndrome. J Hand Surg Am 1994;19:817–20.

43. Rayan GM, Jensen C, Duke J. Elbow flexion test in the normal population. J Hand Surg Am 1992;17: 86–9.

44. Cheng CJ, Mackinnon-Patterson B, Beck JL, et al. The scratch collapse test for evaluation of carpal and cubital tunnel syndrome. J Hand Surg Am 2008;33:1518–24.

45. Mackinnon SE, Novak CB. Compression neuropathies. In: Green DP, Hotchkiss RN, Pederson WC, editors. Green's operative hand surgery, vol. 1, 5th edition. Philadelphia: Elsevier; 2005. p. 999–1045.

46. Gross MS, Gelberman RH. The anatomy of the distal ulnar tunnel. Clin Orthop Relat Res 1985;196: 238–47.

47. de Seze MP, Rezzouk J, de Seze M, et al. Does the motor branch of the long head of the triceps brachii arise from the radial nerve? Surg Radiol Anat 2004; 26:459–61.

48. Prasartritha T, Liupolvanish P, Rojanakit A. A study of the posterior interosseous nerve (PIN) and the radial tunnel in 30 Thai cadavers. J Hand Surg Am 1993; 18:107–12.

49. Ozkan M, Bacakoglu AK, Gul O, et al. Anatomic study of posterior interosseous nerve in the arcade of Frohse. J Shoulder Elbow Surg 1999;8:617–20.

50. Mayer JH, Mayfield PH. Surgery of the posterior interosseous branch of the radial nerve. Surg Gynecol Obstet 1947;84:979.

51. Nielsen HO. Posterior interosseous nerve paralysis caused by fibrous band compression at the supinator muscle: a report of four cases. Acta Orthop Scand 1976;47:304.

52. Riordan DC. Radial nerve paralysis. Orthop Clin North Am 1974;5:283.

53. Sharrard WJ. Posterior interosseous neuritis. J Bone Joint Surg Br 1966;48:777.

54. Spinner M. The arcade of Frohse and its relationship to posterior interosseous nerve paralysis. J Bone Joint Surg Br 1968;50:809.

55. Whitely WH, Alpers BJ. Posterior interosseous palsy with spontaneous neuroma formation. Arch Neurol 1959;1:226.

56. Capener N. The vulnerability of the posterior interosseous nerve of the forearm. J Bone Joint Surg Br 1966;48:770.

57. Capener N. Posterior interosseous nerve lesions. Proceedings of the second hand club. J Bone Joint Surg Br 1964;46:361.

58. Bryan FS, Miller LS, Panijaganond P. Spontaneous paralysis of the posterior interosseous nerve: a case report and review of the literature. Clin Orthop Relat Res 1971;80:9.

59. Woltman HW, Learmonth JR. Progressive paralysis of the nervus interosseous dorsalis. Brain 1934;57:25.

60. Rosenbaum R. Disputed radial tunnel syndrome. Muscle Nerve 1999;22:960–96.

61. Wartenberg R. Cheiralgia parestetica [isolated neuritis of the superficial radial nerve]. Z Ger Neurol Psychiatr 1932;141:145–55 [in German].

62. Dellon AL, Mackinnon SE. Radial sensory nerve entrapment in the forearm. J Hand Surg Am 1986;11:199–205.

Open Versus Endoscopic Carpal Tunnel Release

Dominic J. Mintalucci, MD[a], Charles F. Leinberry Jr, MD[b],*

KEYWORDS

• Carpal tunnel syndrome • Carpal tunnel release • Endoscopic

KEY POINTS

• A solid understanding of the applied surgical anatomy and surface landmarks is preeminent to a successful carpal tunnel release.
• Concerns about the safety and potential increased cost of an endoscopic release have led to the modification of the standard open approach.
• On comparing endoscopic with open carpal tunnel release, there may be some subtle differences; however, both can provide an excellent outcome.

INTRODUCTION

Sir James Paget first described compression of the median nerve at the wrist following a distal radius fracture in 1854.[1] More than 150 years later, carpal tunnel syndrome (CTS) is today the most common compressive disorder in the upper extremity. In 2007, the American Academy of Orthopaedic Surgeons (AAOS) created a clinical practice guideline that defined CTS as a symptomatic compression neuropathy of the median nerve at the level of the wrist, characterized physiologically by evidence of increased pressure within the carpal tunnel and decreased function of the median nerve in the hand.[2]

ANATOMY AND PATHOPHYSIOLOGY

Nine flexor tendons and the median nerve traverse the carpal tunnel, which is bordered dorsally by the concave arch of the carpus, and volarly by the transverse carpal ligament (TCL). The median nerve is the most superficial structure beneath the TCL, and divides into multiple sensory branches and one motor branch after passing through the carpal tunnel.[3] The motor branch, of particular concern during surgical release of the TCL, has been shown to have significant anatomic variation. The motor fascicles arise from the radio-palmar aspect of the nerve in approximately 80% of cases, but may arise centrally or, rarely, ulnarly.[4] Poisel[5] identified 3 major patterns by which the recurrent branch passes through the TCL: extraligamentous, subligamentous, and transligamentous. In his 1977 review of 246 cases, Lanz[6] found the nerve to be extraligamentous in 46%, subligamentous in 31%, and transligamentous in 23% of cases.

Gelberman and colleagues[7] studied the effects of wrist position on interstitial pressure within the carpal tunnel. This study found 2.5 mm Hg to be the normal pressure with the wrist in neutral position, whereas with the wrist in maximal extension and wrist flexion the pressure increased to 30 and 31 mm Hg, respectively. A decrease in epineural blood flow occurs when pressure reaches 20 to 30 mm Hg, and pressures greater than 30 mm Hg diminish nerve conduction.[8] In

Disclosure: All named authors hereby declare that they have no conflicts of interest to disclose related to the topic of this article.
[a] Hand Surgery, Jefferson Medical College, 1025 Walnut Street, Philadelphia, PA 19107, USA; [b] Rothman Institute, Thomas Jefferson University, 925 Chestnut Street, Philadelphia, PA 19107, USA
* Corresponding author.
E-mail address: bikeberry@comcast.net

patients with CTS, interstitial canal pressures were 32 mm Hg in neutral, 94 mm Hg in full flexion, and 110 mm Hg in wrist extension.[7]

DIAGNOSIS

The diagnosis of CTS remains primarily a clinical one, although current trends indicate increased reliance on electrodiagnostic testing (EDX). Nevertheless, as discussed by Bickel,[9] the role of EDX remains unclear. The lack of an appropriate gold-standard test and reliance on EDX testing may lead to the withholding of effective treatment for patients with CTS. To this end, Graham and colleagues[10,11] performed a literature review in 2006 that yielded 6 clinical criteria (CTS-6) proved to correlate positively with a diagnosis of CTS, and stated that the value added by EDX testing was minimal. The 6 clinical criteria are nocturnal numbness, median nerve paresthesia, thenar muscle atrophy, positive Phalen test, positive Tinel test, and loss of 2-point discrimination.

TECHNIQUES OF CARPAL TUNNEL RELEASE

A solid understanding of the applied surgical anatomy and surface landmarks is preeminent to a successful carpal tunnel release. The Kaplan cardinal line correlates to the distal extent of the TCL. It begins with a line drawn at the apex of the first web space, parallel to the proximal palmar crease, and ends just distal to the hook of the hamate.[12] The point where this line intersects with the flexed long finger typically represents the location of the recurrent branch of the median nerve. The palmar cutaneous branch is generally radial to the palmaris longus tendon. A "safe zone" for release may be reproduced by determining the intersection of the longitudinal axis of the flexed ring finger with the distal wrist crease, or alternatively a longitudinal line drawn parallel with the third web space, ending proximally just ulnar to the palmaris longus.

Open carpal tunnel release (OCTR) has long been considered the gold-standard surgical treatment for CTS. The technique involves placement of a longitudinal incision at the base of the hand. The subcutaneous tissue, the superficial palmar fascia, and the muscle of the palmaris brevis (if present) are also incised in line with the incision, thereby exposing the TCL.[13] Scar tenderness, pillar pain, weakness, and delays in return to work can occasionally be seen following an OCTR. These limitations resulted in the development of newer techniques to minimize surgical morbidity and hasten recovery. In 1989, Okutsu and colleagues[14] introduced the concept of an endoscopic carpal tunnel release (ECTR). This landmark technique used a single small incision 3 cm proximal to the wrist crease and released the TCL under direct visualization using a hook knife. In the same year, Chow[15] described a novel ECTR technique using 2 skin incisions. In his report he describes a transbursal approach with one incision just proximal to the wrist flexion crease ulnar to the palmaris longus tendon, and a second longitudinal incision 4 to 5 mm distal to the distal edge of the TCL to allow passage of the endoscope and dissecting instruments superficial to the arch and digital nerves. Agee and colleagues[16] modified the Okutsu technique by also using a single incision but instead used a trigger-deployed blade elevated from the tip of the device. Release of the TCL is performed in a distal to proximal direction.[17] At present many systems are available to perform an ECTR. Furthermore, with the advent of high-definition (HD) monitors and HD arthroscopic cameras, even greater visualization is now possible.

Recently, the standard OCTR has also undergone modifications to minimize surgical morbidity and expedite return to work. These techniques have resulted into what is now referred to as limited-open or mini-open. Lee and colleagues[18] described an approach that attempted to meld the benefits of a minimally invasive release while decreasing the risk of nerve injury. This approach describes a 2.5- to 3.0-cm longitudinal incision placed in line with the radial border of the ring finger or the third web space (although some now only use a 1.5–2.5-cm incision). Dissection is carried to the distal extent of the TCL, and the distalmost aspect of the ligament is incised with a scalpel for approximately 1 cm in a distal to proximal direction, starting ulnar to the midline of ligament. Next a series of instruments are used to create an unimpeded pathway for the passage of a cutting tome device, which bisects the ligament in a distal to proximal direction, resulting in a complete release with preservation of the palmar fascia and palmaris brevis muscle.[19]

COMPARATIVE ANALYSIS OF OPEN VERSUS ENDOSCOPIC CARPAL TUNNEL RELEASE

The debate among hand surgeons in favor of ECTR versus OCTR is as unresolved today as it was during the 1990s. Proponents of both camps cite literature supporting their preferred method, and despite multiple randomized controlled trials no consensus has been reached. The proposed benefit of ECTR versus OCTR is that by dividing the TCL from below, the overlying skin and muscle are preserved, potentially improving postoperative morbidity, facilitating an earlier return to work, and preserving grip strength. Proponents of an open release caution against an increased risk of catastrophic nerve or artery injury owing to limited visualization, a steep learning curve, longer surgical time, and increased cost. In addition, as the paradigm shifts to smaller open incisions, the morbidity associated with the mini-open approaches is potentially lessened.

Return to Work

CTS is one of the most common major disabling workplace injuries, with an incidence of 1 to 3 cases per 1000 subjects per year and a prevalence of 50 cases per 1000 subjects per year.[2] According to the US Bureau of Labor Statistics, in 2005 there was a median loss of 27 workdays with each claim.[20] Foley and colleagues,[21] in their analysis of the economic burden of CTS in Washington State, found that workers recovered only half the preinjury earnings of claimants after 6 years, compared with patients treated for upper extremity fractures during the same period. A Scandinavian study showed a permanent failure to return to work in 11% of CTS claimants,[22] imparting a significant socioeconomic cost to society.

In 2001, Gerristen and colleagues[23] undertook a review of 14 different randomized clinical trials comparing several different surgical techniques for release of the TCL. Included in their review is a section on 7 randomized clinical trials comparing ECTR and OCTR. Their analysis showed slight support with conflicting evidence for an earlier return to work and/or activities of daily living following ECTR, with 4 in favor of ECTR and 3 showing no difference. A 2004 meta-analysis of 13 randomized clinical trials by Thoma and colleagues[24] compared OCTR with ECTR, and analyzed data pooled from 3 studies showing no significant difference between the two techniques.

In 2008, the AAOS published evidence-based guidelines on the treatment of CTS. In its report the Academy specifically addressed pain outcomes, functional status, symptom severity, return to work, grip and pinch strength, infections, wound-related complications, reversible nerve damage, and total complications. Ten studies were identified specifically addressing return to work, 3 of which favored ECTR.[25]

In their 2009 review of the surgical treatment of CTS, the Cochrane Collaboration evaluated a total of 16 studies comparing ECTR with OCTR, and 4 studies comparing minimally invasive OCTR with ECTR. Fourteen studies specifically addressed return to work or activities of daily living, with 8 studies favoring ECTR, 5 showing no difference,

and 1 favoring OCTR. In addition, data were pooled and a meta-analysis provided, based on 3 studies, showing a weighted mean difference in time to return to work as 6 days earlier in the ECTR group.[26]

Short-Term Data

The theoretical benefit of preserving the palmar musculature and skin has not been borne out in the literature. Grip and pinch strength have been used as surrogate measures of overall hand function. Thoma and colleagues[24] performed a meta-analysis pooling 3 randomized clinical trials for outcomes of grip strength, and 2 studies for pinch strength at 12 weeks. The investigators concluded that grip and pinch strength are more likely to be preserved with ECTR at 12 weeks. Data from both this study and that by Gerristen and colleagues[23,24] showed no statistical difference in terms of short-term pain outcomes and short-term symptom relief. Similarly, the AAOS report favored ECTR in terms of pinch strength at 12 weeks. The AAOS also identified 5 studies that evaluated grip strength at 12 weeks with trends favoring ECTR; however, the meta-analysis showed significant heterogeneity, and the investigators were unable to draw a conclusion on differences in functional status at 12 weeks postoperatively.[25] The Cochrane review evaluated short-term data from 11 of 16 studies comparing ECTR with OCTR, 8 of which found no significant difference at 3 months or less. Meta-analysis was performed on 3 studies slightly favoring ECTR in terms of symptom severity scores and functional scores at 12 weeks.[26] In his evidence-based review regarding ECTR versus OCTR, despite inconsistencies in the data, Abrams[27] concluded that the data slightly favor restoration of grip and pinch strength with ECTR. However, these differences have been shown to normalize at 1 year,[28–30] with equivalent outcomes at 5-year follow-up as well.[31]

Complications

Although much of the skepticism surrounding ECTR during its infancy has waned, many still consider endoscopic release to be dangerous secondary to a lack of visualization and concern for nerve or arterial injury. Palmer and Toivonen[32] sent questionnaires on self-reporting any complications following CTR procedures to 1253 members of the American Society for Surgery of the Hand, and received 708 responses regarding ECTR and 616 regarding OCTR. One hundred median nerve injuries, 88 ulnar nerve injuries, 77 digital nerve injuries, and 121 vessel injuries were reported for ECTR. The OCTR respondents reported 147 median nerve injuries, 29 ulnar nerve injuries, 59 digital nerve injuries, and 34 vessel injuries. An alarming number of major complications are thus occurring with both procedures.

Benson and colleagues[33] reviewed 80 publications from 1966 through 2001 yielding 22,327 cases of ECTR and 5669 cases of OCTR. The investigators reported on neuropraxias, and nerve, artery, and tendon injuries. Major nerve injuries were seen in 0.13% compared with 0.10% for ECTR and OCTR patients, respectively. ECTR had a rate of 0.03% for digital nerve injuries and 0.39% for OCTR. Arterial arch injuries occurred in 0.02% of the ECTR group, with no cases in the OCTR group. The most striking difference was in the rate of transient neuropraxias, which were reported in 1.45% of ECTR cases compared with 0.25% of OCTR cases. After exclusion of transient neuropraxia, the rate of major nerve, vessel, or tendon injury was shown to be lower in the ECTR group, at 0.19% compared with 0.49% for the OCTR subset. Similarly, Boecksyns and Sorensen[34] reported a rate of 0.3% for irreversible nerve damage in the ECTR group, and 0.2% for the OCTR group.

Gerristen and colleagues[23] found ECTR to have a higher incidence of transient nerve problems, with OCTR having more wound problems such as infection, hypertrophic scar, and scar tenderness. Thoma and colleagues[24] demonstrated a benefit to ECTR with respect to scar tenderness, but stated that patients were 3 times as likely to experience transient neuropraxia. The AAOS report found 8 studies regarding wound-related complications, with 7 of 8 favoring ECTR. Reversible nerve damage was once again found to be more likely with ECTR, and the AAOS failed to show a statistical difference in terms of general complications or infection.[25] The Cochrane review found no major complications resulting in permanent nerve damage or major impairments, and supported an increased likelihood of transient nerve injury with ECTR and an increase in wound problems (such as infection, hypertrophic scar, and scar tenderness) with OCTR. In addition, they addressed the need for revision surgery. Six studies met criteria for analysis of relative complication risk. Twelve of 513 cases required revision surgery in the ECTR subset versus 5 of 370 OCTR cases.[26]

There would appear to be a relative consensus that major irreversible nerve damage is extremely rare with either procedure, and that both procedures can be performed safely and effectively. There appear to be more wound complications associated with OCTR and more reversible nerve injuries with ECTR. There also appears to be a higher reoperation rate with ECTR.

The Learning Curve

Much has been made about the added cost and time associated with educating hand surgeons regarding ECTR. Despite significant evidence supporting ECTR as a safe and reliable option for release of the TCL, persistent concern about a steep learning curve has been expressed. Macowiec and colleagues[35] addressed this topic in a cadaveric study reviewing the results of ECTR on 573 hands performed in a teaching environment where orthopedic surgeons were being taught the procedure. Incomplete release in 30% of hands was noted using the extrabursal technique and in 42% using the transbursal technique. There were 8 ulnar artery injuries, 7 superficial arch injuries, 2 median nerve injuries, and 1 ulnar nerve injury. The investigators concluded that there is still a significant learning curve in the use of ECTR.

Recently, Beck and colleagues[36] conducted a retrospective review of patients undergoing ECTR by a single surgeon in the first 2 years of practice, comparing results from months 1 to 6, 7 to 12, and 13 to 24 to determine whether a learning curve was present. Results show that during the first 6 months, 8 of 71 ECTRs were converted to OCTR, 1 of 72 were converted during the second 6 months, and 3 of 215 were converted during the second year of practice. No major complications were observed, there was no increase in morbidity for those patients who underwent conversion to OCTR, and there was a 0.28% complication rate in the study. The investigators concluded that despite the presence of a learning curve during the first 6 months of practice, there was no increase in morbidity transferred to the patient.

Cost

Approximately 500,000 carpal tunnel surgeries are performed in the United States annually, costing more than $2 billion per year.[37] Of these, approximately 50,000 are performed endoscopically. Given the huge cost to society, both sides of the debate have cited cost to support their treatment of choice. Chung and colleagues[38] released a cost analysis comparing OCTR with ECTR using quality-adjusted life-years (QALYs). These investigators used 2 randomized clinical trials comparing ECTR with OCTR and derived QALYs from questionnaire results, and concluded that ECTR seemed to be a cost-effective procedure; however, their analysis was extremely sensitive to major complications. As such, their findings may have been biased in favor of ECTR because 1 of the 2 randomized clinical trials had a major nerve complication rate of 1.5% in the OCTR group, compared with 0% for ECTR. However, the incidence of major nerve complications, as discussed earlier, is likely similar when comparing the 2 groups outright.

Vasen and colleagues[39] performed a decision analysis that used a direct cost basis, and applied data to a model using assumptions of risks for complications. Using their model, a complication rate of greater than 6.2% would favor OCTR, a return-to-work difference of less than 21 days would favor OCTR, and a greater than 0.1% incidence of major nerve injury would favor OCTR. The investigators concluded that ECTR was less costly when considering the cost of the procedure and lost wages when using their base assumptions. These base assumptions, however, had several flaws. For one, they assumed a 10-fold increased relative risk of major nerve laceration with ECTR, which has not been borne out in the literature. Furthermore, they failed to factor in any cost associated with a tender scar or pillar pain, and applied an estimate of 365 days of lost wages for any complication encountered (including neuropraxia). This assumption is likely grossly overestimated. In addition, they estimated the difference in return to work between groups to be 28 days, with more recent analysis indicating perhaps only a 6-day improvement in return-to-work outcomes.[26]

Two randomized clinical trials looked directly at surgical costs on comparing OCTR with ECTR. Saw and colleagues[40] estimated an increased cost to ECTR related to initial capital expenditure and the relatively high cost of the single-use blade. These investigators estimated an incremental cost of ECTR to be £98, which was offset by a savings to industry of £67 per day, and an earlier return to work by 8 days. Trumble and colleagues[41] performed a prospective, randomized, multicenter trial on 192 hands in 147 patients. Direct costs were recorded and calculated using surgeon fees, anesthesia fees, cost of equipment (including endoscopic blades), and operating room costs. The mean time from administration of anesthesia to transport from the operating room was 42 minutes for ECTR and 49 minutes for OCTR. The mean cost of OCTR was $3940 compared with $3750 for ECTR. From these results, Trumble and colleagues concluded that there is a significant benefit to ECTR, with not only the direct costs of ECTR being lower but also the indirect cost to society given a 20-day improvement in return-to-work outcomes in the ECTR group.

Mini-Open Versus Endoscopic Carpal Tunnel Release

Concerns about the safety and potential increased cost of an endoscopic release have led to modification of the standard open approach. Theoretically this approach could offer the safety of better visualization of the TCL and an implied decrease in associated neuropraxias seen with the endoscopic approach, while still providing decreased scar tenderness and pillar pain, and better early postoperative grip strength and earlier return to work. Limited data exist that directly compare endoscopic with a minimally invasive open approach; however the Cochrane Collaboration identified 4 studies that directly addressed this comparison.

In their prospective trial, Mackenzie and colleagues[42] reported a slight but significant improvement in early function and comfort, and faster recovery of pinch and grip strength at 2 to 4 weeks, but not at later follow-up in the endoscopic group. Wong and colleagues[43] found improved outcomes in the limited incision group, with improved pain scores at 2 to 4 weeks, no difference in strength, and surprisingly decreased pillar pain at 2 to 4 weeks, but not at later follow-up. Rab and colleagues[44] found no statistically significant difference between the two groups at any time point in terms of grip and pinch strength, hand function, or symptom severity scores. One study favored ECTR in terms of revision surgery, with 1.5% undergoing revision compared with 9% in the modified open-incision group.[45] No studies addressed return to work or activities of daily living.

SUMMARY

Carpal tunnel is a very common hand condition, which after a failure of conservative treatment can be treated successfully with surgical decompression. When comparing ECTR with OCTR there may be some subtle differences; however, both can provide an excellent outcome. Therefore the decision as to which technique should be performed should be left up to the patient and surgeon, depending on his or her training and experience.

REFERENCES

1. Paget J. Lectures on surgical pathology. Philadelphia: Lindsay and Blakiston; 1854.
2. American Academy of Orthopaedic Surgeons Work Group Panel. Clinical guidelines on diagnosis of carpal tunnel syndrome. Available at: www.aaos.org/research/guidelines/CTS_guideline.pdf. Accessed January 30, 2012.

3. Kerwin G, Williams CS, Seiler JG. The pathophysiology of carpal tunnel syndrome. Hand Clin 1996; 12:243–51.

4. Steinberg DR, Szabo RM. Anatomy of the median nerve at the wrist. Open carpal tunnel release—classic. Hand Clin 1996;12:259–69.

5. Poisel S. Ursprung und verlauf des ramus muscularis des nervus digitalis palmaris communis I (n. medianus). Chir Praxis 1974;18:471–4.

6. Lanz U. Anatomical variations of the median nerve in the carpal tunnel. J Hand Surg 1977;2:44–53.

7. Gelberman RH, Hergenroeder PT, Hargens AR, et al. The carpal tunnel syndrome: a study of carpal tunnel pressures. J Bone Joint Surg Am 1981;63: 380–3.

8. Rydevik B, Lundborg G, Bagge U. Effects of graded compression on intraneural blood flow: an in vivo study on rat tibial nerve. J Hand Surg Am 1981;6: 3–12.

9. Bickel KD. Carpal tunnel syndrome. J Hand Surg Am 2010;35:147–52.

10. Graham B, Regehr G, Naglie G, et al. Development and validation of diagnostic criteria for carpal tunnel syndrome. J Hand Surg Am 2006;31:919–24.

11. Graham B. The value added by electrodiagnostic testing in the diagnosis of carpal tunnel syndrome. J Bone Joint Surg Am 2008;90:2587–93.

12. Riordan D, Kaplan E. Surface anatomy of the hand and wrist. In: Spinner M, editor. Kaplan's functional and surgical anatomy of the hand. Philadelphia: JB Lippincott Co; 1984. p. 353–7.

13. Steinberg DR. Surgical release of the carpal tunnel. Hand Clin 2002;18:291–8.

14. Okutsu I, Ninomiya S, Takatori Y, et al. Endoscopic management of carpal tunnel syndrome. Arthroscopy 1989;5:11–8.

15. Chow JC. Endoscopic release of the carpal ligament: a new technique for carpal tunnel syndrome. Arthroscopy 1989;5:19–24.

16. Agee JM, McCarroll HR, Tortosa RD, et al. Endoscopic release of the carpal tunnel: a randomized prospective multicenter study. J Hand Surg Am 1992;17:987–95.

17. Adams B. Endoscopic carpal tunnel release. J Am Acad Orthop Surg 1994;2:179–84.

18. Lee WP, Plancher KD, Strickland JW. Carpal tunnel release with a small palmar incision. Hand Clin 1996;12:271–84.

19. Higgins JP, Graham TJ. Carpal tunnel release via a limited palmar incision. Hand Clin 2002;18: 299–306.

20. US Department of Labor statistics. Updated November, 2011. Available at: www.bls.gov/iif/oshwc/osh/os/osh05_29.pdf. Accessed January 30, 2012.

21. Foley M, Silverstein B, Pollisar N. The economic burden of carpal tunnel syndrome: long term earnings of CTS claimants in Washington State. Am J Ind Med 2007;50:155–72.

22. Bekkelund SI, Pierre-Jerome C, Torbergsen T, et al. Impact of occupational variables in carpal tunnel syndrome. Acta Neurol Scand 2001;103(3):193.

23. Gerritsen AA, Uitdehaag BM, van Geldere D, et al. Systematic review of randomized clinical trials of surgical treatment for carpal tunnel syndrome. Br J Surg 2001;88:1285–95.

24. Thoma A, Veltri K, Haines T, et al. A meta-analysis of randomized controlled trials comparing endoscopic and open carpal tunnel decompression. Plast Reconstr Surg 2004;114:1137–46.

25. Keith J, et al. Treatment of carpal tunnel syndrome. Evidence report. Rosemont (IL): American Academy of Orthopaedic Surgeons; 2008.

26. Scholten RJ, Mink van der Molen A, Uitdehaag BM, et al. Surgical treatment options for carpal tunnel syndrome. Cochrane Database Syst Rev 2009;(4): CD003905.

27. Abrams R. Endoscopic versus open carpal tunnel release. J Hand Surg Am 2009;34:535–9.

28. Ferdinand RD, MacLean JB. Endoscopic versus open carpal tunnel release in bilateral carpal tunnel syndrome. J Bone Joint Surg Br 2002;84:375–9.

29. Atroshi I, Larsson GU, Ornstein E, et al. Outcomes of endoscopic surgery compared with open surgery for carpal tunnel syndrome among employed patients: randomized controlled trial. BMJ 2006; 332:1463–4.

30. MacDermid JC, Richards RS, Roth JH, et al. Endoscopic versus open carpal tunnel release: a randomized trial. J Hand Surg Am 2003;28:475–80.

31. Atroshi I, Hofer M, Larsson GU, et al. Open compared with 2-portal endoscopic carpal tunnel release: a five year follow-up of a randomized controlled trial. J Hand Surg Am 2009;34:266–77.

32. Palmer AK, Toivonen DA. Complications of endoscopic and open carpal tunnel release. J Hand Surg Am 1999;24:561–5.

33. Benson LS, Bare AA, Nagle DJ, et al. Complications of endoscopic and open carpal tunnel release. Arthroscopy 2006;22:919–24.

34. Boecksyns ME, Sorensen AI. Does endoscopic carpal tunnel release have a higher rate of complications than open carpal tunnel release? An analysis of published series. J Hand Surg Br 1999;24:9–15.

35. Makowiec RL, Nagle DJ, Chow JC. Outcome of first-time endoscopic carpal tunnel release in a teaching environment. Arthroscopy 2002;1(18):27–31.

36. Beck JD, Deegan JH, Rhoades D, et al. Results of endoscopic carpal tunnel release relative to surgeon experience with the Agee technique. J Hand Surg Am 2011;36:61–4.

37. Palmer DH, Hanrahan LP. Social and economic costs of carpal tunnel surgery. Instr Course Lect 1995;44:167–72.

38. Chung KC, Walters MR, Greenfield ML, et al. Endoscopic versus open carpal tunnel release: a cost-effective analysis. Plast Reconstr Surg 1998;102:1089–99.

39. Vasen AP, Kuntz KM, Simmons BP, et al. Open versus endoscopic carpal tunnel release: a decision analysis. J Hand Surg Am 1999;24:1109–17.

40. Saw NL, Jones S, Shepstone L, et al. Early outcome and cost-effectiveness of endoscopic versus open carpal tunnel release: a randomized prospective trial. J Hand Surg Br 2003;28B:444–9.

41. Trumble TE, Diao E, Abrams RA, et al. Single portal endoscopic carpal tunnel release compared with open release: a prospective randomized trial. J Bone Joint Surg Am 2002;45:1107–15.

42. Mackenzie DJ, Hainer R, Wheatley MJ. Early recovery after endoscopic vs. short-incision open carpal tunnel release. Ann Plast Surg 2000;44:601–4.

43. Wong KC, Hung LK, Ho PC, et al. Carpal tunnel release: a prospective, randomized study of endoscopic versus limited-open methods. J Bone Joint Surg Br 2003;85:863–8.

44. Rab M, Grunbeck M, Beck H, et al. Intra-individual comparison between open and 2-portal endoscopic release in clinically matched bilateral carpal tunnel syndrome. J Plast Reconstr Aesthet Surg 2006;59:730–6.

45. Eichhorn J, Dieterich K. Open versus endoscopic carpal tunnel release. Results of a prospective study. Chir Praxis 2003;61:279–83 [in German].

Evaluation and Treatment of Failed Carpal Tunnel Release

Valentin Neuhaus, MD, Dimitrios Christoforou, MD,
Thomas Cheriyan, MD, Chaitanya S. Mudgal, MD*

KEYWORDS

- Carpal tunnel release • Evaluation • Failed • Treatment

KEY POINTS

- Treatment failure and complications are encountered in 1% to 25% of all carpal tunnel releases.
- Besides hematoma, infection, skin necrosis, and intraoperative iatrogenic injuries, persistence and recurrence should be included in this discussion. Persistence is often related to incomplete release.
- Operative release is the main treatment for persistence and recurrence consisting of complete decompression of the median nerve. In some circumstances, coverage of the median nerve may be necessary.

INTRODUCTION

Carpal tunnel syndrome (CTS) is the most common compressive peripheral neuropathy of the upper extremity. The annual incidence is approximately 7 cases per 10 000 humans.[1] Carpal tunnel release (CTR) usually provides a good outcome with complete resolution of symptoms. However, treatment failure and complications are encountered in 1% to 25% of all CTR published reports, with a re-operation rate of up to 12%.[2–9]

In 1966, Phalen[10] published his experience of 212 CTRs, with only 2 patients requiring reoperations. He reported that one patient had incomplete severance of the distal portion of the transverse carpal ligament and the second had recurrence caused by scarring.[10]

As described by Phalen and other investigators, the failure of CTR can be classified by the affected or injured structures, the presenting symptoms or complaints, and by the timing of their appearance.[11] Adequate diagnosis and treatment of these failures can be challenging. The definitions and the clinical evidence are yet unclear. They are based only on retrospective studies or small series with anecdotal conclusions. It is also important to note that the terms *recurrence* and *persistence* are typically used interchangeably, which makes analysis of any existing data extremely challenging.

There is a paucity of data specifically addressing recurrent CTS, with many studies purposely excluding patients with recurring symptoms requiring treatment and, furthermore, lacking information regarding the incisions used or subsequent coverage of the median nerve.[12] The authors present a short review that addresses the evaluation and treatment of failed CTR.

COMPLICATIONS AND FAILED TREATMENT OF PRIMARY CTR

The authors distinguish complications based on their timing, namely, intraoperative, early postoperative, and late postoperative complications (**Table 1**).[11] Furthermore, symptoms after failed primary CTR can be classified as persistent, recurrent, or new.

Disclosure: All named authors hereby declare that they have no conflicts of interest to disclose related to this article.

Orthopaedic Hand Service, Massachusetts General Hospital, 55 Fruit Street, Boston, MA 02114, USA
* Corresponding author. Orthopaedic Hand Service, Yawkey Center, Massachusetts General Hospital, 55 Fruit Street, Yawkey Center, Suite 2100, Boston, MA 02114.
E-mail address: cmudgal@partners.org

Orthop Clin N Am 43 (2012) 439–447
http://dx.doi.org/10.1016/j.ocl.2012.07.013

orthopedic.theclinics.com

Table 1
Complications of primary CTR

Intraoperative	Injuries to nerves, vessels, or tendons
Early postoperative	Infection, hematoma, skin necrosis, scar issues, incomplete release of transverse carpal ligament, persistent symptoms
Late postoperative	Complex regional pain syndrome and pillar pain, neuroma formation, scar issues, recurrent or new symptoms

Typically, complications of CTR can arise because of iatrogenic injuries to nerves (palmar cutaneous branch of median nerve, median nerve, and ulnar nerve), vessels, or tendons (including adhesions to the adjacent tissues) as well as bowstringing of the flexor tendons. Pillar pain and complex regional pain syndrome are complications that are not completely understood. Infection, hematoma, skin necrosis, and scar hypertrophy are other additionally reported complications of CTR. Rare complications should also be mentioned, such as pisotriquetral subluxation.[11]

The actual technique of primary CTR does not seem to have an obvious impact on the incidence of complications. Boeckstyns and Sorensen[13] analyzed 54 publications that reported complications of 9516 endoscopic and 1203 open releases. They concluded that endoscopic release was comparable with open release. Although the rate of irreversible nerve damage was similar (0.3% vs 0.2%), they noted that reversible nerve problems were more common after endoscopic release. There was, however, a slightly higher risk of catastrophic complications with endoscopic release, such as complete transection of the median nerve. Tendon lesions were very rare (0.03%); the rate of other complications, such as reflex sympathetic dystrophy, hematoma, or wound problems, was about the same between endoscopic and open CTR.[13]

The main focus of this review is to analyze and discuss the treatment of failed CTR. This treatment can be classified into 2 categories: persistence and recurrence. The clinician must be able to distinguish old from new symptoms, which forms a keystone in distinguishing persistence from recurrence.[14] The rate of revision surgery for persistent or recurrent symptoms has been reported to be 3.1%.[3]

Persistence or transient (less than 6 months)[15] relief of symptoms was often related to incomplete release of the transverse carpal ligament,[16] especially seen with endoscopic techniques.[17,18] In one large series, 54% of all redo-CTRs were caused by incomplete transection of the transverse carpal ligament.[8] Although incomplete release (usually distally,[19] especially in CTR with transverse or short longitudinal incisions) was the most common cause, other causes of persistent or transient symptoms after CTR included tenosynovitis and fibrosis.[20]

In a cadaveric study, Cobb and Cooney[18] showed that carpal arch widening was not affected significantly by the incidence of complete versus incomplete release of the carpal tunnel. They also showed in a clinical study that the outcome of revision surgery was independent of complete versus incomplete release.[21]

An incorrect primary diagnosis can also be a cause for an apparent postoperative persistence of CTS. Conditions like cervical radiculopathy; spinal cord lesions; proximal nerve compressions, such as the pronator syndrome; cervical disk disease; thoracic outlet syndrome; or systemic diseases, such as diabetes mellitus, thyroid disorders, and hemodialysis-related neurologic sequelae, may manifest with symptoms similar to that of CTS.[8,20,22,23] Lesions around the carpal tunnel, like ganglia, arterial aneurysms, gouty tophi, amyloidosis, sarcoidosis, or fracture callus, may compress the median nerve producing symptoms suggestive of CTS.[20] Secondary gain should also be considered in the differential diagnosis.[11]

Recurrent symptoms have been defined as "a significant or complete relief of the patient's original pre-operative symptoms which lasts for a definite period of time after the initial carpal tunnel release, but, eventually, similar symptoms develop again."[15] Jones and colleagues[15] considered 6 months as the minimum symptom-free interval before attributing symptoms to be arising from a recurrence. Possible causes of recurrent symptoms include perineural or intraneural fibrosis (32% of all cases in a large series),[8] scarring, and adherence of the median nerve to adjacent tissue as well as nerve traction with wrist motion caused by adherence, neuroma formation, median nerve subluxation from the carpal tunnel, tenosynovitis, or flexor retinaculum regrowth.[3,24,25] Possible cofactors that have been described include poor hemostasis, excessive period of immobilization, and inappropriate physical therapy.[15] As in patients with persistent symptoms, incomplete release can cause recurrence. Furthermore, less likely causes of recurrence must be kept in mind. For example, there is a case report of an aneurysm of an aberrant median artery causing recurrent symptoms.[19]

New symptoms are usually distinct and can be even more distressing than the primary complaints of the CTS. There are multiple possible causes, including iatrogenic injuries to nerves, vessels, or tendons. Scarring can result in neuromas, fibrosis, and hypertrophic scars leading to neuropathic or pillar pain, dysesthesias, muscle weakness, and stiffness.[15,26,27]

SYMPTOMS AND DIAGNOSIS OF PERSISTENCE AND RECURRENCE

In making the diagnosis and differentiating between persistence and recurrence of CTS, the clinician must perform a thorough history, carefully examine and make a record of the clinical presentation, review the operative report, and possibly use or review additional diagnostic studies. A thorough assessment begins with reviewing the symptoms and, if possible, the electrodiagnostic studies before the primary CTR was performed. Many patients with persistent or recurrent CTS complain of similar symptoms as in primary CTS. Numbness, pain and tingling at night, or even persistent numbness can be present. Physical examination findings, such as weakness of opposition of the thumb or thenar wasting, can also be observed because of long-standing median compression.[21] In persistence, mainly caused by incomplete release (this can also be the cause in recurrence), the symptoms are similar or even unchanged as in primary CTS.[8] In recurrence, they are typically slightly different and accompanied by scar hypersensitivity and oftentimes pain.[28]

Standardized questionnaires for the assessment of severity, functional status, and quality of life in patients who have CTS may be of further value in the assessment after failure of resolution following surgery. These questionnaires have been shown to improve quality of care in the initial surgical management of CTS.[21,29] The consistency of these questionnaires in patients with failed CTR is yet unclear.

The review of the operative report is another essential element in the treatment of patients with failed surgical management of CTS. It encompasses not only what steps were performed but can also offer important hints regarding the individual anatomy.

A thorough clinical examination of both upper extremities as well as the cervical spine follows. The essential components of a thorough evaluation include the inspection of the prior CTR incision and any other scars; sensibility of the median, ulnar, and radial nerves; static and moving 2-point discrimination; grip strength; and provocative testing. Many tests used for the diagnosis of primary CTS can also be used for recurrent or persistent CTS. Among them, the Phalen, Tinel, and Durkan tests are the ones most frequently used.[10,30,31] De Smet[32] published 5 cases with persistent symptoms and concluded that a negative Phalen test and a positive tourniquet (Gilliatt) test can indicate a distally incomplete release of the retinaculum.

All patients with a diagnosis of failed CTR should have further work-up consisting of electrodiagnostic testing to improve accurate diagnosis but also to serve as an objective follow-up parameter. An abnormal electromyogram (EMG) is usually present; however, a normal EMG should not exclude the possibility of persistent/recurrent compressive neuropathy.[28] In addition, it is important to note that electrical changes in EMG can persist for an unpredictable period of time, even after successful CTR.[20] If the clinical signs clearly indicate persistent or recurrent CTS, surgery may be indicated despite a normal EMG. The authors also recommend evaluating bony structures with either a conventional radiograph or even sophisticated imaging, such as an magnetic resonance imaging (MRI) or a computed tomography scan in the case of a posttraumatic presentation to rule out fracture callus or dislocation causing a compression of the median nerve.[33] High-resolution ultrasound may also be be used as an optional resource.[34] Tenosynovitis, any space occupying mass, fibrosis or nerve enhancement can be evaluated. However, it does not seem that MRI can reliably detect incomplete CTR.[33,35] Furthermore, MRI is expensive and the reference standards are not clearly defined.

THERAPY

As already mentioned, the adequate diagnosis and treatment of these failures can be challenging. It is, therefore, essential to make the correct diagnosis of recurrent or persistent CTS. A neuroma of the palmar cutaneous branch of the median nerve is treated with re-exploration of the wound, different from recurrent or persistent CTS. Also, some symptoms should be treated nonoperatively, such as in patients with complex regional pain syndrome.

The next step in management following the accurate diagnosis is the decision of how to treat patients. Nonoperative treatment, such as splinting, injection with local anesthesia or steroids, and activity modification, can be used as a temporizing measure or as a diagnostic tool. However, the data supporting this are lacking. Some investigators prefer to initially try nonsurgical treatment, especially in recurrent CTS.[15,20,36,37] Craft and colleagues[36] recommended microneurolysis and coverage with the hypothenar fat pad flap in recurrent symptoms but only after failed initial nonoperative treatment. In a recently published study, cortisone injection improved the symptoms in 23 out of 28 patients with recurrent CTS.[38] Revision CTR using an extended incision, which crosses the wrist crease into the distal forearm, is the most recommended treatment of persistent or recurrent CTS.[24] Endoscopic release can be a safe treatment in the hands of experienced surgeons but only in cases of late recurrence.[39]

The timing of surgery depends on several factors. Most of the symptoms of numbness and night pain resolve within 24 hours after primary CTR.[40] Jones and colleagues[15] used chronic severe pain for more than 1 year as an indication for revision CTR. However, persistence of numbness for more than 1 year can be present and subsequently resolve in up to 40% patients.[40] O'Malley and his colleagues[19] recommended re-exploration of the carpal tunnel in patients with persistent symptoms causing nocturnal wakening or exacerbated by activities and in those with a positive Phalen test. All of their patients had hypesthesia in the distribution of the median nerve. If incomplete release of the transverse carpal ligament is suspected, a reoperation can be indicated earlier in the course. One large study had an average time of 996 days (range, 15 days to 12 years) between the first and second operation.[8] There is one retrospective study showing no influence on outcome based on the time from the initial operation to the time of revision surgery.[19] The psychological strain of ongoing symptoms on patients can also be used as a helpful guide in timing suitable surgery. However, one must be cautious in attributing too much significance to this because there is always the possibility of secondary gain, poor coping skills, or pain catastrophizing that may exert undue influence not only on the symptom complex but also on the decision-making algorithm of the surgeon, particularly if inexperienced.[41]

In deciding the general operative approach, the main goal of treatment must be exploration of the carpal tunnel in its entirety to completely decompress the median nerve. All persisting fibers of the transverse carpal ligament must be released as well as the antibrachial fascia at the level of the wrist crease and well proximal to it.[15] The exploration, potential external neurolysis, and epineurectomy of the median nerve should be started proximal (from the ulnar side) and distal from the areas that have been scarred to dissect from the known to the unknown anatomy.[20] This procedure is usually done under loupe magnification but may be performed under microscopic magnification. If intrafascicular scarring is significant, internal neurolysis may be considered; however, there is not much data to support this.[24]

Incision

Langloh and Linscheid[6] published their results of 34 re-explorations caused by recurrence in 2053 CTRs. In this series, the carpal tunnel was approached via the previous incision. In 1992, Dellon and Chang[42] presented their series of patients with recurrent CTS. They suggested using an alternative incision for approaching recurrent median nerve compression through unscarred soft tissue, expressing concerns that the median nerve could be intimately associated with or even found within the scar.[42] They used a new incision, which was 1.0 to 1.5 cm ulnar to the prior incision and divided the most ulnar part of the transverse carpal ligament just adjacent to the hook of hamate. They had no complications with a follow-up period of 20 months. Similarly, Mathoulin and colleagues[28] used a linear incision 1 cm away from the original scar along the axis of the fourth finger.

Coverage

Historically, many investigators recommended simple revision nerve decompression depending on the condition of the tissues found intraoperatively.[19,21] More recently, there has been increasing discussion that may support the attempt to create a biologically friendly gliding area for the median nerve. In general, adequate soft tissue coverage of the median nerve is considered to be important. Locally, this is made difficult when there is a significant amount of scarring, which can decrease the ability of the nerve to glide freely. Besides, unlike the ulnar nerve at the elbow, transposition is not an option.

There are several local subcutaneous and muscle flaps that have been described in many articles.[9,25,28,43–46] Varitimidis and colleagues[47] described the use of autogenous saphenous vein wrapping of the median nerve in revision surgery after successful trials in rats. Some investigators indicate that free and pedicled flaps are a superior form of coverage in this setting. Circumferential coverage of the median nerve after neurolysis by a pedicled or free flap of soft tissue might improve the revascularization of the nerve, reduce the traction forces, and improve its gliding capabilities.[24] Described flaps include the lateral arm, hemi-latissimus dorsi muscle, scapular, pedicled reverse radial forearm fascia, and the groin flap.[24,48] The use of a pedicled omentum flap has also been described and can be an alternative in patients who have undergone multiple previous failed surgical procedures.[37]

As discussed by Tollestrup and colleagues,[49] some flaps may be too small to cover the carpal tunnel (palmaris brevis flap, synovial flap), whereas others have potentially high donor site morbidity (abductor digiti minimi [ADQ] flap, pedicled omentum flap) or are technically difficult and require extensive dissection (free flaps). Tham and colleagues[43] also stated that motor loss and bulkiness of some flaps can be limiting. They promote the radial artery fascial flap as another option and reported their results in 6 patients. To reduce scaring and improve nerve gliding, postoperative mobilization should start as soon as possible. However, in the case of a pedicled or free flap, immobilization of the wrist for 10 to 14 days is recommended.[24,50] Some investigators advocate the immobilization of the wrist for 2 to 3 weeks after surgery, even when a flap has not been used.[19,21] Advances in technology now offer alternative coverage options, such as the Canaletto implant (Eurymed, Nimes, France), which is a semirigid silicone and polyethylene implant.[51] In a recent study, the investigators showed good results comparable with other described techniques, avoiding the use of flaps and their associated morbidity.

The Authors' Preferred Choice

If there is a clear reason for persistent or recurrent CTS, such as an incomplete release with adequate tissue left to cover the nerve, the authors proceed with the simple release of the transverse fibers and wound closure. However, if the coverage or surrounding soft tissue bed are in question, the authors prefer coverage with the hypothenar fat pad flap.[49] This flap is technically simple to perform, can be accessed through the same incision, does not influence the function of the hand, provides good covering of the median nerve, and also provides a gliding surface.[49,50] The surgical technique is eloquently described in many articles.[25,28,49,50] The hypothenar fat pad flap receives its vascular supply from the superficial branches of the ulnar artery. If necessary, the deep branch of the ulnar artery near the deep motor branch of the ulnar nerve can be dissected to allow the flap to be mobilized more easily.[28]

Description of the Revision CTR and Coverage with the Hypothenar Fat Pad Flap

Anatomic landmarks are marked out, including the pisiform, the hook of the hamate, Kaplan's cardinal line, and the axis of the ring finger. Thereafter, an incision is made in the base of the palm radial to the axis of the ring finger, if the previous scar is indistinguishable. In cases when the old scar can be easily identified, it is used and is extended across the wrist crease in a Z-shaped fashion and into the distal forearm. After making the initial skin incision, deeper dissection is initially started in the distal forearm to encounter normal tissue identifying the median nerve; from here on out, the median nerve is protected at all times as old scar tissue is encountered. The palmar fascia is opened along the long axis of the limb, and then the transverse carpal ligament is identified. If there is no clear definition to the transverse carpal ligament, dissection is once again started proximally. A Freer elevator is placed deep to the confluence of the transverse carpal ligament and the distal forearm fascia and the dissection proceeds from proximal to distal. Any adhesions of the median nerve to the contents of the carpal tunnel are carefully identified and lysed. Special attention must be paid to adhesions of the median nerve to the undersurface of the transverse carpal ligament or its remnant. The median nerve is decompressed completely. It is often difficult to identify the distal extent of the transverse carpal ligament because of scar formation. The senior author recommends using the sentinel pad of fat as a reliable landmark for having reached the distal most portion of the carpal tunnel. This pad of fat harbors the superficial palmar arch and almost always signifies the distal most extent of the transverse carpal ligament. It is almost always present but may seem atrophic in the very elderly. It is almost always of a darker yellow color than the subcutaneous fat.[52] A hypothenar fat pad flap is then fashioned by undermining the hypothenar skin, dissecting the fat pad, elevating it from its ulnar side but leaving it attached at the radial edge off the palmaris brevis as described by Strickland.[25] An excellent fat pad graft can be acquired in this manner. Dissection in a radial to ulnar direction as the skin is undermined ensures that the fat pad remains well perfused as it receives its perfusion from the radial side. The width of the graft should be adequate to completely cover the median nerve and reach the undersurface of the radial leaf of the transverse carpal ligament. Once this width is determined, the fat pad is divided at its ulnar border and carefully elevated in a radial direction maintaining its radial pedicle. It is then sewn to the undersurface of the radial leaf of the transverse carpal ligament to cover the median nerve but should avoid any tension in the graft to minimize any chance of compression from it (**Fig. 1**). In situations when the quality of the local tissues is

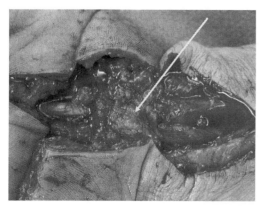

Fig. 1. Intraoperative appearance of the median nerve covered with a hypothenar fat pad flap (*yellow arrow*).

suboptimal and scarring of the hypothenar fat pad is either suspected preoperatively or evident during surgery, the senior author prefers using the ADQ to cover the median nerve.[44,53] It is important to alert patients and obtain their consent preoperatively regarding the possibility of using the ADQ. The bulk of the ADQ after transfer provides a well-perfused muscle cover for the nerve but can preclude direct wound closure (**Figs. 2–4**). A split-thickness skin graft is then used for skin coverage over the transferred muscle. Great care must be taken to maintain the integrity of the vascular pedicle of the ADQ at its base. In most circumstances, however, the hypothenar fat pad flap is available and affective for coverage and use of the ADQ flap is extremely

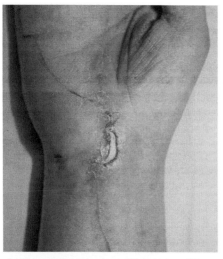

Fig. 2. This patient had multiple operations with wound breakdown over a synthetic mesh. The quality of the local tissue was suboptimal; therefore, an ADQ flap was chosen. Note the preoperative incision marking.

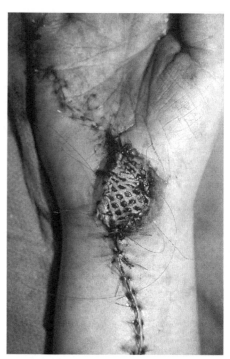

Fig. 3. After complete release of the median nerve, the nerve was covered with an ADQ flap. The bulky flap precluded direct wound closure. A split-thickness skin graft was then used for coverage of the dehiscent area.

uncommon. After a routine closure, the patients' upper limb is placed in a splint. Digital motion is encouraged from the day of surgery. After 1 week, the authors discontinue the splint and start a range-of-motion program for the wrist (see **Fig. 3**). If a split-thickness skin graft has been used, the authors continue immobilization for 10 to 12 days before starting a range-of-motion program.

OUTCOME OF RECURRENT SURGERY AND COMPLICATIONS

Outcomes of recurrent surgery can vary. Some studies report relatively poor results, with up to 95% of patients complaining of persisting symptoms.[54] Other reports indicate that 60% to 70% of patients consider themselves cured or improved, with the remaining 30% to 40% describing their condition as unchanged or worse.[19,48] In some of these unsatisfied patients, other diagnoses, such as cervical radiculopathy, seemed to be a contributing factor.[19] Strickland and colleagues[25] reported an overall satisfaction rate of 95%.[25] One study suggested that an incomplete release found at revision surgery likely has the best prognosis, whereas fibrosis correlated with a poor

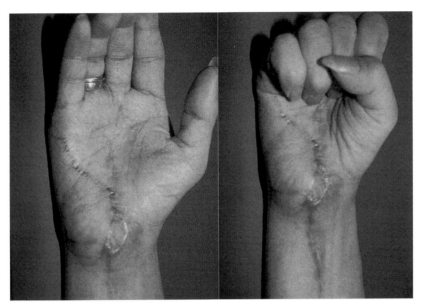

Fig. 4. Aesthetic and functional outcome. (*Courtesy of* Chaitanya Mudgal, MD.)

outcome.[19] This finding is also consistent with the findings of Hulsizer and colleagues[55] who showed that the outcome of revision surgery was better in patients having undergone primary endoscopic treatment, assuming incomplete release was the reason for failed treatment.

The results of steroid injection in patients with recurrent CTS coupled with physical examination findings has been shown to provide a good screening test to predict the outcome following recurrent surgery.[38] Cobb and colleagues[21] pointed out that abnormal preoperative nerve conduction studies were associated with a significantly better outcome than patients with normal EMGs. However, they could not find any significant difference in outcomes between patients who had incomplete versus complete previous release.[54]

Postoperative complications include (superficial) wound complications and complex regional pain syndrome in 10% to 30%.[19,37] Donor site problems are often encountered, such as abnormal sensation, itching, or aesthetically disturbing scars.[48]

Symptomatic Relief

Jones and colleagues[24] showed that epineurectomy with circumferential wrapping of a flap around a scarred median nerve significantly improved the subjective pain rating in 3 out of 4 patients. Recurrent CTS treated with external neurolysis and coverage with the hypothenar fat pad flap resulted in 91% (41 out of 45) resolution of pain.[28] Dahlin and colleagues[48] presented even

better results: 13 out of 14 patients had significantly less pain and improved sensation and reduced numbness. Another study reported symptomatic relief in all patients after endoscopic CTS without any complications.[39]

Functional Recovery

Chang and Dellon[56] presented their results of 35 recurrent CTR operations with an early postoperative mobilization protocol in 30 patients. The sensorimotor function, assessed with a numerical score from 0 to 10, improved significantly.[56]

In another study whereby nearly 80% of patients had a positive Phalen sign before revision surgery, most patients improved significantly, with only 18% having a persistent Phalen sign after revision surgery.[25] The Tinel sign disappeared in 26 out of 28 patients and 43 out of 45 patients with recurrent CTS after microneurolysis and coverage with a -hypothenar fat pad flap, respectively.[28,36] In addition, the 2-point discrimination and the grip strength improved, but this was not statistically significant.[25]

Several studies suggest worker's compensation may serve as a confounding variable resulting in a poorer reported outcome as has been demonstrated in primary CTS.[57] Concannon and colleagues[4] presented a higher recurrence rate after endoscopic CTR in patients on worker's compensation. Strasberg and colleagues[54] also showed that a patient's chance of a successful outcome was significantly less in patients on worker's compensation. In addition, there was a trend toward a worse outcome in older women.

SUMMARY

Treatment failure and complications are encountered in 1% to 25% of all CTRs. Besides hematoma, infection or skin necrosis, and intraoperative iatrogenic injuries, persistence and recurrence should be included in this discussion. Persistence is often related to incomplete release. Similar symptoms recurring after a symptom-free interval of 6 months are considered recurrent and may be caused by intraneural or perineural scarring. Adequate diagnosis and treatment of these failures can be challenging. Operative release is the main treatment consisting of complete decompression of the median nerve. In some circumstances, coverage of the median nerve may be necessary. The authors' preferred treatment of choice is the hypothenar fat pad flap, which is technically simple and has good, reproducible results. However, 30% to 40% of patients may still be unsatisfied with the outcome.

REFERENCES

1. Jenkins PJ, Watts AC, Duckworth AD, et al. Socioeconomic deprivation and the epidemiology of carpal tunnel syndrome. J Hand Surg Eur Vol 2012;37(2):123–9.

2. Bande S, De Smet L, Fabry G. The results of carpal tunnel release: open versus endoscopic technique. J Hand Surg Br 1994;19(1):14–7.

3. Cobb TK, Amadio PC. Reoperation for carpal tunnel syndrome. Hand Clin 1996;12(2):313–23.

4. Concannon MJ, Brownfield ML, Puckett CL. The incidence of recurrence after endoscopic carpal tunnel release. Plast Reconstr Surg 2000;105(5):1662–5.

5. Kulick RG. Carpal tunnel syndrome. Orthop Clin North Am 1996;27(2):345–54.

6. Langloh ND, Linscheid RL. Recurrent and unrelieved carpal-tunnel syndrome. Clin Orthop Relat Res 1972;83:41–7.

7. Murphy RX Jr, Jennings JF, Wukich DK. Major neurovascular complications of endoscopic carpal tunnel release. J Hand Surg Am 1994;19(1):114–8.

8. Stutz N, Gohritz A, van Schoonhoven J, et al. Revision surgery after carpal tunnel release–analysis of the pathology in 200 cases during a 2 year period. J Hand Surg Br 2006;31(1):68–71.

9. Wulle C. Treatment of recurrence of the carpal tunnel syndrome. Ann Chir Main 1987;6(3):203–9.

10. Phalen GS. The carpal-tunnel syndrome. Seventeen years' experience in diagnosis and treatment of six hundred fifty-four hands. J Bone Joint Surg Am 1966;48(2):211–28.

11. Akelman E. Carpal tunnel syndrome. In: Richard A, Berger AP, editors. Hand surgery, vol. 1. Philadelphia: Lippincott Williams & Wilkins; 2004. p. 867–85.

12. Brown RA, Gelberman RH, Seiler JG 3rd, et al. Carpal tunnel release. A prospective, randomized assessment of open and endoscopic methods. J Bone Joint Surg Am 1993;75(9):1265–75.

13. Boeckstyns ME, Sorensen AI. Does endoscopic carpal tunnel release have a higher rate of complications than open carpal tunnel release? An analysis of published series. J Hand Surg Br 1999; 24(1):9–15.

14. Tung TH, Mackinnon SE. Secondary carpal tunnel surgery. Plast Reconstr Surg 2001;107(7):1830–43 [quiz: 44,933].

15. Jones NF, Ahn H, Eo S. Revision surgery for persistent and recurrent carpal tunnel syndrome and for failed carpal tunnel release. Plast Reconstr Surg 2011;129(3):683–92.

16. Kulick MI, Gordillo G, Javidi T, et al. Long-term analysis of patients having surgical treatment for carpal tunnel syndrome. J Hand Surg Am 1986;11(1):59–66.

17. Forman DL, Watson HK, Caulfield KA, et al. Persistent or recurrent carpal tunnel syndrome following prior endoscopic carpal tunnel release. J Hand Surg Am 1998;23(6):1010–4.

18. Cobb TK, Cooney WP. Significance of incomplete release of the distal portion of the flexor retinaculum. Implications for endoscopic carpal tunnel surgery. J Hand Surg Br 1994;19(3):283–5.

19. O'Malley MJ, Evanoff M, Terrono AL, et al. Factors that determine reexploration treatment of carpal tunnel syndrome. J Hand Surg Am 1992;17(4):638–41.

20. Steyers CM. Recurrent carpal tunnel syndrome. Hand Clin 2002;18(2):339–45.

21. Cobb TK, Amadio PC, Leatherwood DF, et al. Outcome of reoperation for carpal tunnel syndrome. J Hand Surg Am 1996;21(3):347–56.

22. Yamauchi K. A recurrent case of carpal tunnel syndrome in haemodialysis. Hand Surg 2002;7(2):299–303.

23. Eason SY, Belsole RJ, Greene TL. Carpal tunnel release: analysis of suboptimal results. J Hand Surg Br 1985;10(3):365–9.

24. Amadio PC. Interventions for recurrent/persistent carpal tunnel syndrome after carpal tunnel release. J Hand Surg Am 2009;34(7):1320–2.

25. Strickland JW, Idler RS, Lourie GM, et al. The hypothenar fat pad flap for management of recalcitrant carpal tunnel syndrome. J Hand Surg Am 1996; 21(5):840–8.

26. Palmer AK, Toivonen DA. Complications of endoscopic and open carpal tunnel release. J Hand Surg Am 1999;24(3):561–5.

27. Louis DS, Greene TL, Noellert RC. Complications of carpal tunnel surgery. J Neurosurg 1985;62(3):352–6.

28. Mathoulin C, Bahm J, Roukoz S. Pedicled hypothenar fat flap for median nerve coverage in recalcitrant carpal tunnel syndrome. Hand Surg 2000;5(1):33–40.

29. Levine DW, Simmons BP, Koris MJ, et al. A self-administered questionnaire for the assessment of severity of symptoms and functional status in carpal tunnel syndrome. J Bone Joint Surg Am 1993; 75(11):1585–92.

30. Durkan JA. A new diagnostic test for carpal tunnel syndrome. J Bone Joint Surg Am 1991;73(4):535–8.

31. Stewart JD, Eisen A. Tinel's sign and the carpal tunnel syndrome. Br Med J 1978;2(6145):1125–6.

32. De Smet L. Recurrent carpal tunnel syndrome. Clinical testing indicating incomplete section of the flexor retinaculum. J Hand Surg Br 1993; 18(2):189.

33. Campagna R, Pessis E, Feydy A, et al. MRI assessment of recurrent carpal tunnel syndrome after open surgical release of the median nerve. AJR Am J Roentgenol 2009;193(3):644–50.

34. El Miedany YM, Aty SA, Ashour S. Ultrasonography versus nerve conduction study in patients with carpal tunnel syndrome: substantive or complementary tests? Rheumatology (Oxford) 2004;43(7):887–95.

35. Wu HT, Schweitzer ME, Culp RW. Potential MR signs of recurrent carpal tunnel syndrome: initial experience. J Comput Assist Tomogr 2004;28(6):860–4.

36. Craft RO, Duncan SF, Smith AA. Management of recurrent carpal tunnel syndrome with microneurolysis and the hypothenar fat pad flap. Hand (N Y) 2007;2(3):85–9.

37. Goitz RJ, Steichen JB. Microvascular omental transfer for the treatment of severe recurrent median neuritis of the wrist: a long-term follow-up. Plast Reconstr Surg 2005;115(1):163–71.

38. Beck JD, Brothers JG, Maloney PJ, et al. Predicting the outcome of revision carpal tunnel release. J Hand Surg Am 2012;37(2):282–7.

39. Teoh LC, Tan PL. Endoscopic carpal tunnel release for recurrent carpal tunnel syndrome after previous open release. Hand Surg 2004;9(2):235–9.

40. Gilbert MS, Robinson A, Baez A, et al. Carpal tunnel syndrome in patients who are receiving long-term renal hemodialysis. J Bone Joint Surg Am 1988; 70(8):1145–53.

41. Cowan J, Makanji H, Mudgal C, et al. Determinants of return to work after carpal tunnel release. J Hand Surg Am 2012;37(1):18–27.

42. Dellon AL, Chang BW. An alternative incision for approaching recurrent median nerve compression at the wrist. Plast Reconstr Surg 1992;89(3):576–8.

43. Tham SK, Ireland DC, Riccio M, et al. Reverse radial artery fascial flap: a treatment for the chronically scarred median nerve in recurrent carpal tunnel syndrome. J Hand Surg Am 1996;21(5):849–54.

44. Leslie BM, Ruby LK. Coverage of a carpal tunnel wound dehiscence with the abductor digiti minimi muscle flap. J Hand Surg Am 1988;13(1):36–9.

45. Dellon AL, Mackinnon SE. The pronator quadratus muscle flap. J Hand Surg Am 1984;9(3):423–7.

46. Rose EH, Norris MS, Kowalski TA, et al. Palmaris brevis turnover flap as an adjunct to internal neurolysis of the chronically scarred median nerve in recurrent carpal tunnel syndrome. J Hand Surg Am 1991;16(2):191–201.

47. Varitimidis SE, Riano F, Vardakas DG, et al. Recurrent compressive neuropathy of the median nerve at the wrist: treatment with autogenous saphenous vein wrapping. J Hand Surg Br 2000;25(3):271–5.

48. Dahlin LB, Lekholm C, Kardum P, et al. Coverage of the median nerve with free and pedicled flaps for the treatment of recurrent severe carpal tunnel syndrome. Scand J Plast Reconstr Surg Hand Surg 2002;36(3):172–6.

49. Tollestrup T, Berg C, Netscher D. Management of distal traumatic median nerve painful neuromas and of recurrent carpal tunnel syndrome: hypothenar fat pad flap. J Hand Surg Am 2010;35(6): 1010–4.

50. Chrysopoulo MT, Greenberg JA, Kleinman WB. The hypothenar fat pad transposition flap: a modified surgical technique. Tech Hand Up Extrem Surg 2006;10(3):150–6.

51. Bilasy A, Facca S, Gouzou S, et al. Canaletto implant in revision surgery for carpal tunnel syndrome: 21 case series. J Hand Surg Eur Vol 2012;37(7):682–9.

52. Madhav TJ, To P, Stern PJ. The palmar fat pad is a reliable intraoperative landmark during carpal tunnel release. J Hand Surg Am 2009;34(7): 1204–9.

53. Cirrincione C, Stern PJ. The abductor digiti minimi muscle flap: an adjunct in the treatment of metacarpal osteomyelitis. J Hand Surg Am 1991;16(5): 824–7.

54. Strasberg SR, Novak CB, Mackinnon SE, et al. Subjective and employment outcome following secondary carpal tunnel surgery. Ann Plast Surg 1994;32(5):485–9.

55. Hulsizer DL, Staebler MP, Weiss AP, et al. The results of revision carpal tunnel release following previous open versus endoscopic surgery. J Hand Surg Am 1998;23(5):865–9.

56. Chang B, Dellon AL. Surgical management of recurrent carpal tunnel syndrome. J Hand Surg Br 1993; 18(4):467–70.

57. Cotton P. Symptoms may return after carpal tunnel surgery. JAMA 1991;265(15):1922–5.

Late Reconstruction of Median Nerve Palsy

Jia-Wei Kevin Ko, MD, Adam J. Mirarchi, MD*

KEYWORDS

- Median nerve injury • Tendon transfer • Nerve palsy • Thenar reconstruction • Opponensplasty

KEY POINTS

- Median nerve injuries are classified as low and high and many more options exist for low median nerve palsies.
- Restoration of thumb opposition is the main goal of reconstructive surgery.
- Successful tendon transfers recreate thumb opposition, which involves 3 basic movements: thumb abduction, flexion, and pronation.
- Loss of sensation to the median aspect of the hand is a relative contraindication to tendon transfer.

INTRODUCTION

Median nerve palsy is arguably one of the most debilitating injuries to the hand, particularly if the ability to achieve thumb opposition is lost. Most reconstructive operations for late median nerve palsies are aimed at restoration of motor function and thumb opposition. Outcomes of any late reconstruction are often dictated by the amount of sensation that has been restored. Median nerve palsies are classified as "high" or "low" based on their anatomic location. Many reconstructive options exist but are limited by the location of the lesion and other associated injuries.

ANATOMY

The median nerve arises from the medial and lateral cords of the brachial plexus. It does not give off any motor or sensory branches until it courses distal to the cubital fossa. At this point, the nerve pierces and innervates the 2 heads of the pronator teres muscle. In the forearm, the median nerve travels between flexor digitorum superficialis (FDS) and the flexor digitorum profundus (FDP) muscle bellies. Motor branches extend to FDS, flexor carpi radialis, and palmaris longus. A major motor branch, the anterior interosseous nerve (AIN), separates to innervate flexor pollicis longus (FPL), pronator quadratus, and FDP to the index and long fingers. The palmar cutaneous nerve branches off in the forearm approximately 5 cm proximal to the wrist flexion crease, providing sensation to the radial aspect of the palm. The remaining nerve travels through the carpal tunnel, where the recurrent motor branch innervates the intrinsic thenar muscles, including abductor pollicis brevis (APB), opponens pollicis, and the superficial head of flexor pollicis brevis (FPB). The deep head of the FPB is innervated by the ulnar nerve. Additional median motor branches innervate the lumbricals of the index and middle fingers. Sensory branches exiting distal to the carpal tunnel provide sensation to volar aspect of the thumb, index, middle, and radial half of the ring fingers.

CLASSIFICATION

The classification of median nerve palsies is based on the anatomic location of the lesion.

Low median nerve palsies are typically described as lesions that occur distal to the origin

Department of Orhtopedics, Oregon Health and Science University, Portland, OR, USA
* Corresponding author.
E-mail address: ajm3874@yahoo.com

Orthop Clin N Am 43 (2012) 449–457
http://dx.doi.org/10.1016/j.ocl.2012.07.014

of the AIN. Functionally, this affects the thenar musculature and median innervated intrinsic, resulting in loss of thumb opposition and sensory loss in the median nerve distribution as described earlier. In part, because the FPB has duel innervation from both the median and the ulnar nerve, not all patients with isolated median nerve palsy will experience complete loss of thumb opposition.

High median nerve palsies are lesions that occur proximal to the origin of the AIN. In addition to potentially creating the same motor and sensory deficits as low median nerve injuries, high median nerve lesions affect the muscles of the forearm. Functionally, this results in diminished forearm pronation from denervation of the pronator teres and pronator quadratus and loss of thumb interphalangeal (IP) joint flexion from denervation of FPL. Patients can also experience wrist flexion weakness from denervation of the flexor carpi radialis and grip strength as a result of the denervation of FDS and FDP to the index and middle fingers. High median nerve lesions are more functionally debilitating and difficult to recover from. They also have implications for the potential reconstructive options for median nerve palsies given their greater functional deficits.

CAUSES

There are many causes of median nerve palsies, and they can broadly be characterized into traumatic, compressive, congenital, and other diseases affecting sensory and motor function. Traumatic causes include direct nerve laceration or contusion and brachial plexus injuries. Compressive causes most commonly include carpal tunnel and radiculopathy from nerve root compression. Although it is not technically considered a palsy, congenital absence of the thenar muscles can result in similar functional deficits as median nerve lesions and require similar reconstructive operations. Many other diseases can affect median nerve function, including Charcot-Marie-Tooth, leprosy, syringomyelia, spinal muscular atrophy, Guillain-Barre, and polio. Although it is currently more of historical interest, polio was once considered to be the most ideal indication for reconstructive opponensplasty for median nerve palsy because it is purely a motor deficit.

INDICATION FOR SURGERY

Most reconstructive options that are currently used for late median nerve palsy are aimed at the restoration of thumb opposition. As noted, because of variations in anatomy and the patient's ability to compensate, functional loss of opposition

is not present in all median nerve palsies, even when the nerve is completely transected. Jensen reported that opponensplasty was needed in only 14% of the patients he encountered.[1] Additionally, loss of thumb opposition may not present a large functional barrier for some patients, particularly if they have low functional demands or the deficit involves the nondominant hand.

If a nerve deficit results from a direct laceration, direct repair or grafting should be the first line of treatment. This may allow for sufficient functional recovery such that reconstruction is not needed and provides the best chance for sensation to be restored. In cases whereby direct repair is not possible or functional loss of opposition remains despite repair, reconstructive surgery may be indicated. It should be noted that permanent sensory loss might compromise the functional outcome of any reconstructive operation even if it is technically successful.[2] Therefore, some surgeons consider loss of thumb sensibility to be a relative contraindication to reconstructive surgery. However, others have advocated for early surgery despite sensory loss, noting that tendon transfers serve as internal splints and eyesight compensates for sensory loss.[3]

In addition to these considerations, the general principles of tendon transfer must be respected.[4] The importance of these basic principles of tendon transfer cannot be overstated and will ensure optimal clinical outcomes. They are listed here:

1. A tendon transfer should not be performed in the presence of an unhealed wound.
2. The full passive joint motion must be restored before tendon transfer.
3. Transfer should not pass through areas of scar tissue or under skin grafts, and surgical incisions should not be placed directly over the transfer.
4. Cutaneous sensation should be restored before the tendon transfer, if possible.
5. The normal function of the transferred muscle must be expendable.
6. The transferred muscle must be under voluntary control and have an independent action.
7. The transferred muscle must have sufficient amplitude and power to perform its new function; thus, reinnervated muscles should be used only in exceptional circumstances.
8. If the transfer cannot perform its new function with a straight line of pull from its origin to its insertion, it should pass through no more than one pulley. Acute angulation of the transfer at the pulley should be avoided.
9. Synergism between the muscle's original and new actions facilitates rehabilitation.

PRINCIPLES OF OPPONENSPLASTY

The mechanics of thumb opposition involves 3 basic movements: thumb abduction, flexion, and pronation. The APB primarily drives opposition, although there is some modest contribution from the opponens pollicis and FPB.[2] In 1938, Bunnell published the essential principles of opponensplasty that complement the general principles of tendon transfer.[5] First, he noted that the direction of pull of a transferred tendon should be from the direction of the pisiform bone. Second, he stated that the insertion of the tendon transfer should be on the dorsoulnar aspect of the proximal phalanx of the thumb so that the transfer can more accurately restore thumb pronation. These principles are still generally adhered to today although the distal insertion site now used for most tendon transfers is at the dorsoradial aspect of the proximal phalanx near the anatomic insertion of the APB tendon and thumb extensor expansion. More recent studies have demonstrated that adequate thumb pronation is still achieved with this insertion site.[6–8]

SPECIFIC OPPONENSPLASTIES FOR LATE MEDIAN NERVE PALSIES
Bunnell Opponensplasty (Ring Finger FDS Transfer)

The ring finger FDS tendon transfer was originally conceived by Royle in 1938.[9] In his original description, the ring FDS tendon was detached from its insertion site on the middle phalanx, retrieved via a secondary incision at the wrist flexion crease, and rerouted through the FPL tendon sheath. Thompson later modified this technique in 1942 so that the ring FDS tendon was rerouted subcutaneously to the thumb base instead of through the FPL tendon sheath.[10] It was later appreciated that detaching the FDS tendon from its insertion site made the proximal IP joint prone to contractures and swan neck deformities.[11] The current recommendation is that the tendon be harvested between the A1 and A2 pulley near the metacarpophalangeal (MP) joint.

Bunnell was the first to describe the technique most commonly used today in which a slip of the flexor carpi ulnaris (FCU) tendon is used to create a fixed pulley for the ring FDS tendon to pass through.[5] This creates a direction of pull near the pisiform as previously noted. Other pulley sites have also been proposed, including the angle at the distal edge of the flexor retinaculum, Guyon canal, and the ulnar border of the palmar aponeurosis.[7] Multiple possible pulley site options allow the surgeon to customize a transfer to address a patient's specific functional deficit. Pulley sites near the pisiform produce the most thumb abduction and opposition, whereas pulley sites distal to this increase the amount of thumb MP joint flexion that can be achieved.[2]

The surgical technique involves first releasing the ring FDS tendon distally, most commonly between the A1 and A2 pulley. A secondary incision is then made just proximal to the wrist crease over the FCU tendon. A distally based radial slip of the FCU tendon is created, leaving about 4 cm of tendon attached to its insertion on the pisiform. A distally based slip has been shown to best prevent pulley migration.[12] The proximal end of the slip is used to create a loop (pulley) and is sewn to itself at the distal insertion on the pisiform (**Fig. 1**). A third incision is made over the dorsal aspect of the thumb MP joint. A subcutaneous tunnel is developed from the loop to the thumb incision to

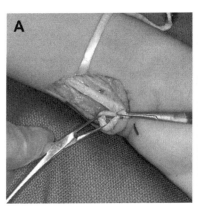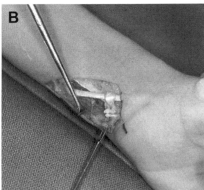

Fig. 1. (*A, B*) A distally based pulley is created using a slip of the FCU tendon, through which the ring FDS tendon is passed through to create a direction of pull near the pisiform bone to recreate optimal opposition. (*Courtesy of Shriners Hospital for Children, Philadelphia, PA.*)

allow passage of the ring FDS. The tendon is passed through the tunnel and inserted into a bone tunnel on the dorsoulnar aspect of the base of proximal phalanx. This is Bunnell's original description, although other insertion sites, such as suturing to the APB tendon insertion without making a bone tunnel, can also be used. Tensioning of the tendon transfer is critical and must be set such that the thumb is fully opposed when the wrist is in a neutral position.

The ring finger FDS serves as an excellent option for tendon transfer because there is sufficient tendon length to reach the base of the thumb and the muscle has good motor strength. However, in higher median nerve lesions, FDS function may be compromised. There is also a small loss in grip strength from sacrificing the ring FDS tendon, although clinically debilitating deficits are typically rare. In traumatic situations, the proximity of the FDS to the median nerve makes it susceptible to concurrent injury. Therefore, careful examination should be conducted before considering the use of this tendon for transfer.

Burkhalter Opponensplasty (Extensor Indicis Proprius Transfer)

The extensor indicis proprius (EIP) tendon transfer was originally described by Burkhalter and colleagues in 1973.[13] Extensor tendons were not initially considered acceptable for restoration of thumb opposition because of their relative weakness and the long course needed to route the tendon to its insertion site. The EIP transfer was developed out of a need for a transfer option in patients in whom the finger flexors were not available to be used. Combined ulnar and median nerve lesions or high median nerve lesions are classic examples.

To perform this procedure, the EIP tendon is transected distally at the level of the MP joint of the index finger along with a slip of the extensor hood. The defect in the hood must be carefully repaired; otherwise, extensor lag may develop from subluxation of the extensor mechanism. Some have argued that extending the functional tendon length by including a slip of the extensor hood is not typically needed, although the tendon is usually just long enough to reach its intended insertion.[14] The tendon is mobilized to a longitudinal incision over the dorsoulnar aspect of the distal forearm (**Fig. 2**A). Occasionally, an additional small incision needs to be created more distally on the dorsum of the hand to help free soft tissue attachments, which may prevent mobilization. Any tissue adherent to the EIP muscle belly is freed to increase tendon excursion. The tendon is then passed subcutaneously to a small incision just proximal to the pisiform. Finally, the tendon is passed to an incision over the APB

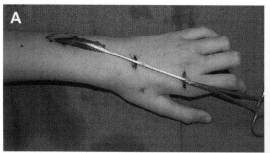
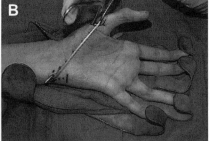
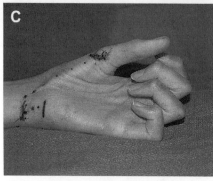

Fig. 2. (*A*) The EIP tendon is harvested from the dorsum of the index MP joint and mobilized to an incision over the dorsoulnar aspect of the distal forearm. (*B, C*) The tendon is mobilized to the palmar aspect of the hand and passed through a subcutaneous tunnel to its insertion site on the base of the thumb. (*Reprinted from* Jones NF, Machado GR. Tendon transfers for radial, median, and ulnar nerve injuries: current surgical techniques. Clin Plast Surg 2011;38(4):621–42.)

insertion, its final anchor point (see **Fig. 2**B and C). The transferred tendon is tensioned and sutured in place with the wrist held in 30° of flexion and the thumb fully opposed.

Once complete, wrist extension should produce some thumb abduction, and wrist flexion should produce some thumb adduction through a tenodesis effect. Excessive thumb extension or flexion with wrist extension may be an indication that the tendon was fixed too dorsally or volarly, respectively.[15] One of the main drawbacks of this procedure is that EIP has weak motor function. However, this transfer is attractive because there is little disability from using the EIP tendon as a donor. This characteristic is making it increasingly popular, even for low median nerve palsies.

Camitz Opponensplasty (Palmaris Longus Transfer)

The Camitz opponensplasty is one of the earliest described tendon transfers for the restoration of thumb opposition.[16] This simple transfer has the benefit of little donor site morbidity because of the extraneous function of the palmaris longus tendon. This transfer is most commonly performed in elderly patients with functional deficits resulting from chronic carpal tunnel syndrome. This transfer can be performed in conjunction with a carpal tunnel release while awaiting median nerve function to return.[17] The presence of a palmaris longus tendon must be confirmed before the procedure.

The procedure is performed by making an incision over the palmaris longus tendon distal to the wrist crease, roughly in line with the web space between the middle and ring fingers (**Fig. 3**A). Because the palmaris tendon is not long enough to reach the base of the thumb, the functional tendon length is increased by harvesting a strip of palmar fascia in line with the distal palmaris longus tendon (see **Fig. 3**B). The tendon is passed through a subcutaneous tunnel over to the base of the thumb and sewn to the insertion of the APB tendon. The tendon is tensioned with the thumb in full opposition and the wrist in a neutral position.

Although this transfer adequately restores thumb abduction, it is less successful at reproducing thumb pronation or flexion because the direction of tendon pull is not from the region of the pisiform (see **Fig. 3**C). The palmar cutaneous nerve is also at risk with the incision, although this risk can be minimized by cheating the incision more ulnarly at the level of the wrist crease. The palmaris tendon is also unavailable for use in high median nerve lesions and can easily be injured in traumatic median nerve injuries given its superficial location and proximity to the nerve.

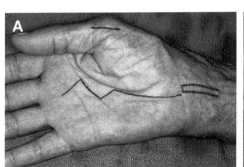
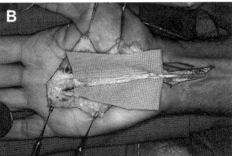
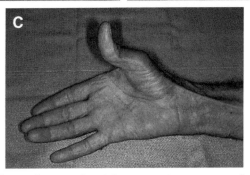

Fig. 3. (*A*) Typical incision used to perform a palmaris longus tendon opponensplasty. (*B*) A strip of palmar fascia is harvested in line with the distal end of the palmaris longus tendon in provide enough length to reach the base of the thumb. (*C*) Although thumb abduction is typically restored, pronation and flexion are difficult to achieve with this transfer given its direction of pull. (*Reprinted from* Jones NF, Machado GR. Tendon transfers for radial, median, and ulnar nerve injuries: current surgical techniques. Clin Plast Surg 2011;38(4):621–42.)

Nevertheless, this transfer can be an effective option in the appropriate patient.

Huber Opponensplasty (Abductor Digiti Minimi Transfer)

This technique was originally described by Huber in 1921[18] and is the earliest tendon transfer described to restore opposition. Because the abductor digiti minimi (ADM) is innervated by the ulnar nerve, this transfer can be used in both low and high median nerve palsies. This procedure is also unique in that it is one of the more cosmetically appealing transfers because it restores bulk to the thenar eminence. It is particularly useful in cases of severe atrophy or when there is congenital absence of the thenar muscles.

The incision for this procedure begins over the pisiform and extends distally and ulnarly toward the insertion of the ADM near the ulnar border of the small finger proximal phalanx (**Fig. 4**A). The ADM tendon is detached from its distal insertion site. It is then carefully released from all of its adjacent soft tissue attachment proximally toward its origin on the pisiform (see **Fig. 4**B). Care must be taken to protect the neurovascular pedicle supplying the ADM muscle. The neurovascular pedicle is typically located on the deep surface of the muscle belly, closer to its proximal origin on the pisiform. Huber's original description left the proximal ADM insertion attached to the pisiform. Littler and Cooley modified this by detaching the ADM tendon from its proximal origin but leaving it in continuity with a slip of the distal FCU tendon.[19] This modification allows for increased tendon excursion because there is usually just enough tendon length to reach the base of the thumb. Ogino and colleagues described another technique if additional tendon length is required. In their modification, the proximal origin of ADM is detached from the pisiform and reattached to the palmaris longus tendon.[20] Others have described a variation in which no formal reattachment of the proximal tendon origin is performed.[21] Further mobilization of the ADM muscle is not without risk, however, because greater mobilization places more tension on the neurovascular bundle. As in other transfers, the distal end of the tendon is attached to the insertion of the APB tendon. The tendon is tensioned with the thumb in full opposition.

This procedure is technically more difficult than some of the other procedures described. Therefore, it has been suggested that it should be used only if other tendon transfers are unavailable. Its most widespread use is in pediatric patients who have congenital absence of their thenar muscles.

Phalen and Miller Opponensplasty (Extensor Carpi Ulnaris Transfer)

The extensor carpi ulnaris (ECU) transfer was originally developed to reconstruct thumb opposition in instances when the wrist and finger flexors were unavailable for transfer.[22] In the original series reported by Phalen and Miller, this was most often a result of combined median and ulnar nerve injuries and when there was extensive muscle damage to the forearm flexors resulting from trauma. Their technique was the first to describe the use of the ECU tendon without the need for free tendon grafting.

This procedure is performed by first isolating the extensor pollicis brevis (EPB) tendon. A small incision is made over the dorsoradial border of the distal forearm. The EPB tendon is identified and transected proximally at its musculotendinous

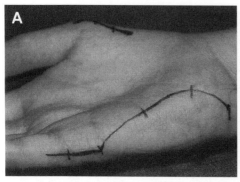
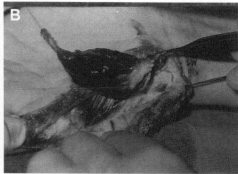

Fig. 4. (*A*) Typical incisions used to perform an ADM opponensplasty. (*B*) The ADM muscle is carefully mobilized back toward its origin on the pisiform, being ever mindful to protect the neurovascular pedicle. (*From* Cawrse NH, Sammut D. A modification in technique of abductor digiti minimi [Huber] opponensplasty. J Hand Surg Br 2003;28(3):233–7; with permission.)

junction to preserve as much tendon length as possible. A secondary incision is made over the dorsum of the thumb MP joint near the insertion of the EPB tendon. The transected EPB tendon is passed distally into this incision. The distal insertion site of the EPB tendon on the dorsal surface of the thumb proximal phalanx is preserved. If a slip exists between the EPB and EPL tendons, it must be divided; otherwise, thumb IP joint extension may be inadvertently occur.[2] Next, an "L"-type incision is made on the ulnar border of the distal forearm, crossing transversely over the volar wrist crease to expose as far radially as the palmaris tendon. The ECU tendon is transected as far distally as possible near its insertion site on the base of the fifth metacarpal. The ECU tendon is freed from its soft tissue attachments proximally, including removal of the tendon from its extensor compartment. The free tendon ends of the EPB and ECU are passed toward each other subcutaneously across the volar aspect of the palm and sewn together.

This tendon transfer may be useful in specific instances when other tendon transfers are unavailable. However, the EPB tendon is sometimes absent in some anatomic variations. Additionally, there have been reports of radial deviation deformities at the wrist affecting grip strength following this transfer.[23]

Schneider Opponensplasty (Extensor Digiti Minimi Transfer)

Inspired by the work of Phalen and Miller with the use of forearm extensors for opponensplasty, Schneider conceived using extensor digiti minimi (EDM) as an additional option for opponensplasty when the forearm flexors are unavailable.[24] This procedure may be useful in instances when the EIP is unavailable for transfer. To perform this procedure, the presence of an EDM must be confirmed. Independent extension of the small finger while the remaining fingers are flexed at the MP joint confirms presence of the EDM.

A small incision is made over the dorsum of the MP joint of the small finger. If a slip from EDC exists to the small finger, it must be identified and preserved. The EDM tendon is identified and released distally from its insertion on the common extensor hood. There are often 2 or more slips of the EDM tendon, and all of them must be released. The extensor hood is then repaired to prevent extensor lag. The tendon is brought proximally to an incision on the dorsoulnar aspect of the distal forearm. The tendon is withdrawn through the extensor retinaculum and freed from its more proximal soft tissue attachments. A subcutaneous tunnel is then developed across the palmar aspect

of the hand to the base of the thumb. The tendon is passed through this tunnel and attached to the ADM tendon with the thumb in full opposition.

This transfer provides yet another option for a surgeon when the other, more common transfers are unavailable. The EDM tendon is typically just long enough to reach its insertion site, so harvesting an additional slip of the extensor hood in continuity with the EDM tendon may be prudent. However, taking more of the extensor hood also increases the risk for extensor lag. Although less commonly performed than some of the other transfers described, Schneider reported good thumb in 8 of 10 patients in his original series.

Postoperative Care After Opponensplasty

In general, the thumb should be immobilized in an opposed position for a minimum of 3 weeks following surgery. The thumb IP joint is typically immobilized in extension, especially if the tendon transfer is inserted onto the APB tendon and common extensor expansion, as is most commonly done. The wrist must also be immobilized in any tendon transfers that involve tendons that cross the wrist joint. Following removal of the splint, early rehabilitation typically focuses on wrist motion, which passively moves and stresses the tendon transfer insertion on the thumb in most of the transfers described. Gradual progression to active motion and neuromuscular training can then begin under guidance of a hand therapist. In certain higher-risk instances, such as when sensation is compromised or in combined median and ulnar nerve lesions, further protective splinting has been advocated to restrict thumb adduction, supination, and extension for up to 3 months.[2]

Specific Considerations for High Median Nerve Palsies

In addition to affecting the intrinsic muscles of the thumb, high median nerve palsies also affect the extrinsic muscles in the forearm. High traumatic median nerve lacerations have a high rate of recovery of the forearm musculature following nerve repair.[2] However, if recovery of extrinsic muscle function is not anticipated, surgical intervention may be warranted.

The loss of forearm pronation is not commonly addressed surgically because this typically does not present a significant functional impairment for the patient. Regrettably, there are few good reconstructive options available for restoring forearm pronation. Loss of thumb and index finger flexion can also persist after high median nerve lesions. Although these do not reliably produce a profound function deficit, some reconstructive options have been described for patients when it does.

For restoration of index finger flexion, an extensor carpi radialis longus to index FDS transfer has been described. Alternatively the index FDS can be sewn in a side-to-side fashion to the common FDS tendon.[2] For restoration of thumb flexion, a brachioradialis to FPL transfer has been described.[2] Excessive tensioning for both of these transfers must be avoided to prevent flexion contractures from developing. Both of these transfers must only be performed across supple joints because of the limited excursion of the transferred muscles. Also, if transfers for extrinsic muscle deficits are performed early, as has been advocated in the past, it is important to perform them in an end-to-side or side-to-side fashion so that any functional recovery of the native motor function is not compromised.[3]

Restoration of thumb opposition in high median nerve injuries adheres to the techniques described earlier here. In general, the EIP, EDM, ADM, and ECU can all be considered for transfer. However, there is a lower likelihood that sensation will return in high median nerve palsies. Therefore, although reconstruction options may be feasible, they may do little to improve a patient's function.

Restoration of Sensation in Median Nerve Palsies

Restoration of sensation in late median nerve palsies remains a challenge. This is particularly true for high median nerve lesions, which have a lower rate of sensory recovery than low median nerve lesions. If sensation is not returned following direct nerve repair grafting, there are few surgical options to address this. Historically, neurovascular skin island transfers have been attempted.[25] However, these have largely been abandoned because of issues with erroneous localization and double sensation phenomenon.[26] More recently, sensory nerve transfer has been attempted and shown to have good success in restoring protective sensation.[27,28]

Nerve Transfers for Median Nerve Palsies

Some of the newest techniques described to address median nerve palsies are nerve transfers. Nerve transfers carry the theoretical advantage over tendon transfers because they do not require prolonged immobilization and muscles remain in their native location. Hsiao has described a technique to address a high median nerve palsies.[29] In this procedure, extrinsic motor function was restored through the transfer of the motor branch of the extensor carpi radialis brevis to the motor branch for pronator teres, and the motor branch to the supinator was transferred to AIN. Nerve transfers must be performed within 12 to 18 months of the original injury, before degeneration of the motor end plates. This technically demanding technique is new but may represent an option for certain patient populations.

SUMMARY

Median nerve palsies can result in debilitating functional deficits to patients, and higher lesions typically present a greater barrier to function and recovery. Several surgical options are available to address many of these deficits, particularly thumb opposition, but the resultant functionality of the hand is often most closely related to its sensibility. Optimal surgical intervention is patient specific and dependent on the unique functional deficit and tendons available for transfer. Newer nerve transfer techniques for both sensory and motor restoration have shown promise but are not yet widely used.

REFERENCES

1. Jensen EG. Restoration of opposition of the thumb. Hand 1978;10(2):161–7.
2. Davis TR. Median and ulnar nerve palsy. In: Wolfe S, Hotchkiss RN, Pederson WC, et al, editors. Green's operative hand surgery. Philadelphia: Elsevier; 2011.
3. Burkhalter WE. Early tendon transfer in upper extremity peripheral nerve injury. Clin Orthop Relat Res 1974;104:68–79.
4. Beasley RW. Principles of tendon transfer. Orthop Clin North Am 1970;1(2):433–8.
5. Bunnell S. Opposition of the thumb. J Bone Joint Surg Am 1938;20(2):269–84.
6. Cooney WP, Linscheid RL, An KN. Opposition of the thumb: an anatomic and biomechanical study of tendon transfers. J Hand Surg Am 1984;9(6):777–86.
7. Lee DH, Oakes JE, Ferlic RJ. Tendon transfers for thumb opposition: a biomechanical study of pulley location and two insertion sites. J Hand Surg Am 2003;28(6):1002–8.
8. Roach SS. Biomechanical evaluation of thumb opposition transfer insertion sites. J Hand Surg Am 2001;26(2):354–61.
9. Royle ND. An operation for paralysis of the thumb intrinsic muscles of the thumb. JAMA 1938;111:612–3.
10. Thompson T. A modified operation for opponens paralysis. J Bone Joint Surg Am 1942;26:632–40.
11. North ER, Littler JW. Transferring the flexor superficialis tendon: technical considerations in the prevention of proximal interphalangeal joint disability. J Hand Surg Am 1980;5(5):498–501.

12. Sakellarides HT. Modified pulley for opponens tendon transfer. J Bone Joint Surg Am 1970;52(1):178–9.

13. Burkhalter W, Christensen RC, Brown P. Extensor indicis proprius opponensplasty. J Bone Joint Surg Am 1973;55(4):725–32.

14. Posner MA, Kapila D. Restoration of opposition. Hand Clin 2012;28(1):27–44.

15. Jones NF, Machado GR. Tendon transfers for radial, median, and ulnar nerve injuries: current surgical techniques. Clin Plast Surg 2011;38(4):621–42.

16. Camitz H. Uber die behandlung der oppositionslahmung. Acta Orthop Scand 1929;65:77–81.

17. Littler JW, Li CS. Primary restoration of thumb opposition with median nerve decompression. Plast Reconstr Surg 1967;39(1):74–5.

18. Huber E. Hilfsoperation bei median uhlahmung. Dtsch Arch Klin Med 1921;136:271.

19. Littler JW, Cooley SG. Opposition of the thumb and its restoration by abductor digiti quinti transfer. J Bone Joint Surg Am 1963;45:1389–96.

20. Ogino T, Minami A, Fukuda K. Abductor digiti minimi opponensplasty in hypoplastic thumb. J Hand Surg Br 1986;11(3):372–7.

21. Cawrse NH, Sammut D. A modification in technique of abductor digiti minimi (Huber) opponensplasty. J Hand Surg Br 2003;28(3):233–7.

22. Phalen GS, Miller RC. The transfer of wrist extensor muscles to restore or reinforce flexion power of the fingers and opposition of the thumb. J Bone Joint Surg Am 1947;29(4):993–7.

23. Wood VE, Adams J. Complications of opponensplasty with transfer of extensor carpi ulnaris to extensor pollicis brevis. J Hand Surg Am 1984;9(5):699–704.

24. Schneider LH. Opponensplasty using the extensor digiti minimi. J Bone Joint Surg Am 1969;51(7):1297–302.

25. Tubiana R, Duparc J. Restoration of sensibility in the hand by neurovascular skin island transfer. J Bone Joint Surg 1961;43B:474–80.

26. Oka Y. Sensory function of the neurovascular island flap in thumb reconstruction: comparison of original and modified procedures. J Hand Surg Am 2000;25(4):637–43.

27. Brunelli GA. Sensory nerves transfers. J Hand Surg Br 2004;29(6):557–62.

28. Bertelli JA, Ghizoni MF. Very distal sensory nerve transfers in high median nerve lesions. J Hand Surg Am 2011;36(3):387–93.

29. Hsiao EC. Motor nerve transfers to restore extrinsic median nerve function: case report. Hand (N Y) 2009;4(1):92–7.

Acute Carpal Tunnel Syndrome

Rick Tosti, MD[a], Asif M. Ilyas, MD[b,c],*

KEYWORDS

- Acute carpal tunnel syndrome • Median neuropathy • Distal radius fracture • Wrist trauma

KEY POINTS

- Acute carpal tunnel syndrome is characterized by rapid onset of median neuropathy caused by sudden increases in carpal tunnel pressures, which leads to ischemia of the median nerve.
- The most common cause is traumatic injury, although atraumatic sources should also be recognized.
- Patients generally complain of pain, lose two-point discrimination, and may demonstrate elevated compartment pressure on measurement.
- Prompt recognition and surgical decompression are imperative to spare median nerve viability.

INTRODUCTION

Carpal tunnel syndrome is a well-known compressive neuropathy of the median nerve characterized by chronic progression of pain and numbness over the radial 3.5 digits and thenar atrophy. If left untreated, advanced stages may result in permanent deficits.[1,2] Rarely, adverse events or risk factors such as trauma, swelling, infections, inflammation, anomalous anatomy, coagulopathy, or tumors may acutely raise intracanal pressure and produce the same constellation of signs and symptoms but with rapid progression. In such cases, the rate and severity at which symptoms progress and the potential for devastating and lasting effects distinguish acute carpal tunnel syndrome (ACTS) as an important clinical entity.[3–7]

ANATOMY

The carpal tunnel is an hourglass-shaped conduit through which nine flexor tendons and the median nerve traverse to gain entry into the hand. With the exception of the transverse carpal ligament (TCL) volarly, the canal is otherwise surrounded by the bones of the carpus, which form the floor (dorsally) and the walls (radially and ulnarly).

Grossly, the inlet of the carpal tunnel can be approximated by the volar wrist crease and the outlet is marked by Kaplan's cardinal line. Cross-sectional investigations by Cobb and colleagues[8] have shown that the width of the tunnel proximally and distally is roughly 25 mm, whereas the narrowest region (at the level of the hamate) averages 20 mm. The depth has been measured at 12 to 13 mm at the proximal and distal ends, whereas the narrow region between the thickest part of TCL and prominent capitate is about 10 mm. The total volume is estimated to be 5 mL.[9]

The TCL is suspended from the scaphoid and trapezium radially and the hamate and pisiform ulnarly. Just deep to the TCL, the most superficial structure is the median nerve, which usually courses just radial to the midline. The median nerve supplies the sensation the radial 3.5 digits, the thenar musculature, and the lumbricals of the index and middle fingers. Generally, the motor fascicles face the radial side. Specifically, the recurrent motor branch of the median nerve innervates the thenar compartment and has a variable anatomy,

Disclosure: All named authors hereby declare that they have no conflicts of interest to disclose related to the topic of this article.

a Orthopaedic Surgery, Temple University Hospital, Philadelphia, PA, USA; b Hand & Upper Extremity Surgery, Rothman Institute, 925 Chestnut Street, Philadelphia, PA 19107, USA; c Orthopaedic Surgery, Thomas Jefferson University, Philadelphia, PA, USA
* Corresponding author.
E-mail address: asif.ilyas@rothmaninstitute.com

Orthop Clin N Am 43 (2012) 459–465
http://dx.doi.org/10.1016/j.ocl.2012.07.015
0030-5898/12/$ – see front matter © 2012 Elsevier Inc. All rights reserved.

which has been described as extraligamentous (branching after the carpal tunnel), subligamentous (branching within the carpal tunnel), and transligamentous (piercing the TCL).[10] The remaining contents of the canal include the four tendons of flexor digitorum superficialis and the four tendons of the flexor digitorum profundus, which are encapsulated by the ulnar bursa, and the flexor pollicis longus, which is encapsulated in the radial bursa.

PATHOPHYSIOLOGY

The possible inciting events leading to ACTS are innumerable and include a variety of traumatic, hematologic, rheumatologic, anatomic, homeostatic, and infectious causes. However, the final common pathway seems to converge with the following sequence of events: a space-occupying lesion creates a mass effect, which increases intracanal pressures. The carpal tunnel behaves like a closed compartment, because the circumferential bony and ligamentous architecture are unyielding and further bounded by occlusive synovial tissue at the entry and exit. As the pressures increase to a threshold level, perfusion of the epineurium decreases and this causes ischemia. Tissue ischemia leads to nerve conduction block, endoneurial edema, and dysfunction of axonal transport, which manifest as the classic symptoms along the median nerve territory.[4] Experiments in animal models have shown a dose–response relationship correlating the duration and severity of exposure to the level of nerve dysfunction and ability to recover.[11] Case series have corroborated this assertion by citing permanent nerve damage in unrecognized or delayed cases.[7,12]

CAUSES

Although considered a rare entity, a large number of case reports have described ACTS originating from a variety of sources. Traumatic injury causing hemorrhage remains the most common mechanism (**Fig. 1**).[2,6,7] However, an assortment of atraumatic causes is not uncommon (see later discussion) . A comprehensive list of factors precipitating ACTS was gathered from case reports and is listed in **Table 1**.

ACTS resulting from a distal radius fracture is the most classically described mechanism. The first description of carpal tunnel syndrome by Paget in 1853 involves median nerve compression following a distal radius fracture that "repaired by an excessive quantity of new bone."[13] Although the details of the onset or progression of median neuropathy in Paget's patient are unknown, many reviews have reported distal radial fractures

as a cause since the distinction between acute and chronic CTS was further defined. Frykman[14] reported the incidence of ACTS following distal radius fractures ranges as 2.3%. However, subsequent authors have cited ranges from 0.2% to 21.3% percent.[5] Following this injury, the mechanism leading to ACTS is hemorrhage into the carpal tunnel or the deep distal forearm at the fracture site.[15]

In a retrospective case-control study, Ring and colleagues investigated risk factors that may herald impending ACTS and found that only fracture displacement was predictive. However, a threshold risk (as a percentage of translation) was only defined in one subgroup: females younger than 48 years old with greater than 35% translation. Other risk factors, such as age, gender, inclination, dorsal tilt, mechanism of injury, ipsilateral injury, or open wound were not significant risk factors.[16]

Case reports have demonstrated that carpal bone fractures, dislocations, and fracture-dislocations have been implicated in the development of ACTS. Among those listed are injuries to the scaphoid, hamate and triquetrum, trapezoid, metacarpals, carpometacarpal joints, and transscaphoid perilunate dislocations. Furthermore, lacerations, burns, animal bites, and high-pressure injection injuries have necessitated carpal tunnel release in some patients.[3,17]

Traumatic iatrogenic causes also deserve special consideration. Edema and hematoma formation following elective and traumatic surgery, excessive injection into the carpal tunnel for reduction, and hyper-flexion of the wrist in an external fixator or the Cotton-Loder position following reduction of a distal radius fracture are preventable insults that should be avoided.

Atraumatic

Numerous atraumatic causes have been described and most of the literature consists of rare case reports. Numerous fluids and space-occupying lesions, such as bleeding, edema, purulence, tumors, and inflammatory pathologies, are possible causes.

Bleeding into the carpal tunnel or intraneural hematoma may occur in persons receiving anticoagulation, hemophiliacs, or those with von Willebrand disease.[18–20] Edematous states may also raise intracanal pressures; examples include pregnancy, burns, venom and toxins, and pancreatic transplant recipients, who experience fluid shifts as a result of intraneural electrolyte imbalances following normalization of their diabetic state.[6,21–23] Infections such as intracarpal canal sepsis, metacarpal osteomyelitis, worms, mycobacterium leprae

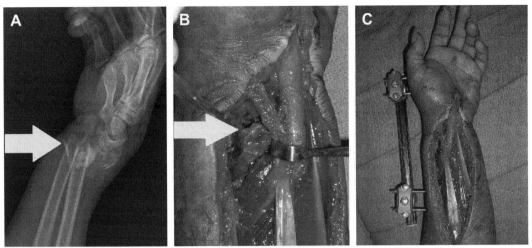

Fig. 1. Distal radius fractures are the most common cause of an ACTS. (*A*) Comminuted distal radius with extensive dorsal displacement (*yellow arrow*) with a large cortical fragment angulated volarly. The patient presented with excruciating pain in the wrist and numbness in the radial 3.5 digits. (*B*) Volar cortical fragments (*yellow arrow*) displaced in this position can apply direct pressure on the median nerve as it enters the carpal tunnel. (*C*) Enlarged hemorrhagic condition of the median nerve on the postreduction image following gross fracture reduction and decompression of the carpal tunnel and the volar forearm fascia.

abscesses, or infectious flexor tenosynovitis directly create an expansive purulent fluid within the carpal tunnel; whereas parvovirus, upper respiratory tract infections, or septic arthritis may raise canal pressures by adjacent intraarticular effusions and synovitis.[24–30] Similarly, inflammatory arthritis or aggressive overuse can irritate the synovium and compress the median nerve.[6,31–33]

Solid lesions may additionally create a mass effect. Tumors are probably the most obvious space-occupying lesion, whereas anatomic anomalies may be more difficult to diagnose. One of the most commonly cited anatomic variants is the persistent median artery, which can become symptomatic secondary to thrombosis, calcification, aneurysm, or hemorrhage.[34–37] Anomalous

Table 1
Causes of acute carpal tunnel syndrome

Trauma	Infection	Inflammatory
Distal radius fracture	Infectious tenosynovitis	Excessive overuse
Metacarpal fracture	Septic arthritis	(flexor synovitis)
Carpal bone fracture	Cellulitis	Pseudogout
Scaphoid dislocation	Filarial infection	Gout
Lunate dislocation	Metacarpal osteomyelitis	Calcifying tendinitis
Perilunate dislocation	Parvovirus	Hydroxyapatite deposition
High-pressure injection	Toxic shock syndrome	Alendronic acid deposition
Laceration	Intracarpal canal sepsis	Rheumatoid arthritis
Animal bite	Leprosy	
Tumor		**Coagulopathy**
Giant cell tumor		Hemophilia
Hemangioma	**ACTS**	von Willebrand disease
Myxofibrosarcoma		Warfarin
Iatrogenic	**Fluid shift**	**Anatomy**
Surgical hematoma	Burns	Anomalous lumbricals
Hyperflexion after external fixation	Stonefish toxin	Median artery thrombosis
Cotton-Loder position	Snake venom	Median artery aneurysm
Tumescent fluid	Pregnancy	Median artery rupture
	Pancreas transplant	Venous malformation

muscle bellies from the flexor tendons or lumbricals have also been described.[38] Finally, solid deposits of minerals, such as alendronic acid or calcium, from gout or pseudogout, may additionally crowd the potential space.[31,32,39]

DIAGNOSIS
History and Physical Examination

In general, the diagnosis of ACTS is a clinical one. History-taking should focus on identifying the risk factors and possible causes previously discussed herein, and it should recognize any preexisting conditions such as diabetic or alcoholic neuropathy, which may confuse the physical examination. The onset of symptoms is on the order of hours to days following an initiating event. Patients will complain of pain and numbness over the median nerve distribution, and progressive stages may reveal weakness, which can be tested by the strength of the abductor pollicis brevis muscle. Two-point discrimination is probably the most useful physical examination maneuver. Mack and colleagues[5] defined an abnormal distance as greater than 15 mm. Bauman and colleagues[7] noted that patients initially were able to distinguish two points less than 6 mm but, by 6 to 12 hours, those with ACTS could not discriminate points greater than 20 mm. The temporal relationship noted by Bauman and colleagues[7] is an important one to distinguish ACTS from nerve contusion or neurapraxia. The patient should have a documented normal examination at the time of presentation and progressively develop paresthesia. In contrast, nerve contusion or neurapraxia presents initially with paresthesia, which improves (or does not progress) over time. Another important differential is that of forearm or hand compartment syndrome, which presents as pain out of proportion with passive stretch and a firm compartment palpated over the forearm or hand with elevated intracompartmental pressures on measurement. The distribution of dysesthesias may be more global in the late stages of compartment syndrome because the ulnar and dorsal sensory radial nerves may be additionally compromised.

Imaging

Musculoskeletal imaging can be a useful adjunct in the diagnosis of ACTS to evaluate for underlying fracture, dislocations, or masses of the wrist. Standard orthogonal radiographs of the wrist, hand, and forearm should always be obtained. CT scan, MRI, and bone scans may provide useful information if the cause remains unclear. However, these tests are generally not available in the emergency setting and may delay definitive treatment.

Pressure Monitoring

Mack and colleagues[5] advocated the routine use of intratunnel pressure monitoring in the diagnosis of ACTS. In their case series, they suggested the following algorithm: in patients with objective sensory deficits, a trial of conservative management is reasonable. If relief is not provided after 2 hours following reduction, splinting, and elevation, then intracarpal pressure monitoring can be considered. The technique involves introduction of a wick catheter into the carpal tunnel via a starting point 1 cm proximal to the distal wrist crease. The needle is directed at a 45° angle heading distally (**Fig. 2**), advanced until the bony carpus is engaged, and then drawn back 0.5 cm. A normal individual measures approximately 1 to 4 mm Hg with the wrist in neutral position; flexion or extension will elevate the measurement.[7] Lundborg and colleagues[40] described a critical threshold of 40 mm Hg—above which nerve ischemia is imminent. In a subsequent study, Szabo and colleagues[41] also suggested median nerve damage was a function of ischemia, which occurred when canal pressures were within 30 mm Hg of the diastolic blood pressure. By externally applying a pressure to the wrist and measuring with a wick catheter, they noted threshold pressures of 60 to 70 mm Hg for patients in whom diastolic blood pressures exceeded 90 mm Hg. A modified algorithm for management of acute median neuropathy is seen in **Fig. 3**.

TREATMENT

Open decompression of the carpal tunnel is the treatment of choice for ACTS. In patients with distal radius fractures with normal appearing carpal tunnels, Lewis[15] suggested extending the proximal incision an additional 4 in to evacuate

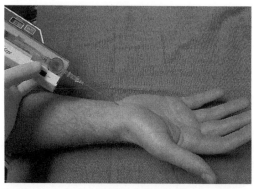

Fig. 2. The pressure monitor enters the carpal tunnel at a 45° angle in line with the ring finger. The starting point is 1 cm proximal to the wrist crease.

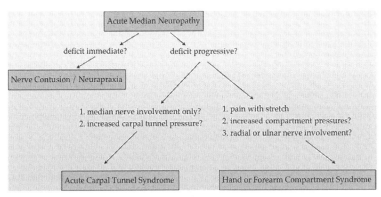

Fig. 3. Differential diagnosis of acute median neuropathy.

hematoma from the fracture site beneath the deep forearm fascia. Furthermore, an extended sigmoid incision may also be made to accommodate internal fixation at the time of decompression. Atraumatic cases should also be treated with appropriate medical management. Adamson and colleagues[6] described successful management of a pregnant woman with splinting, elevation, and diuretics. Management of bleeding diatheses is controversial: hemophiliacs are traditionally given a trial of conservative management, including factor VIII replacement, splinting, and elevation. The optimal observation time is unknown, and it seems that surgery is generally required to resolve the symptoms.[19] Other bleeding conditions, such as warfarin therapy or von Willebrand disease, have been successfully managed surgically without the addition of clotting factors, vitamin K, or fresh frozen plasma.[18,20] ACTS secondary to inflammatory disorders or mineral deposits may benefit from a tenosynovectomy, in addition to releasing the TCL, and soft tissue masses should be sent for open biopsy. Infectious causes may require multiple irrigations and debridements, and the wound is usually left partially open to drain. Anomalous anatomic structures are rare. Dickinson and Kleinert[35] recommended resection of a persistent median artery if perfusion of the hand remains normal after clamping the median artery and releasing the tourniquet. Accessory muscle bellies in the carpal tunnel can be freed from crowding the nerve.[38]

OUTCOMES

Prompt recognition and decompression of ACTS can result in full recovery of the nerve; although the severity and duration of symptoms follow a dose-response curve in the experimental model.[11] It seems that a greater duration or severity corresponds to a greater time to recovery if full recovery is even achievable. Clinically, the dose-response phenomenon was demonstrated in case series by Bauman and colleagues,[7] and by Ford and Ali,[12] who showed that delayed intervention of only 36 to 96 hours, in some cases, had permanent consequences. Furthermore, Adamson and colleagues[6] also reported recovery on within weeks for patients who experienced weeks of symptoms. The optimal time to decompression to avoid permanent deficits is not defined. In an experimental model, Lundborg[42] demonstrated increasing nerve dysfunction and edema after approximately 8 hours of ischemic time. Mack and colleagues[5] cited the Lundborg[42] study as the justification for immediate decompression within 8 hours in their series on patients with ACTS. Consequently, four of five patients treated with urgent decompression experienced full recovery by 96 hours status after carpal tunnel release.

SUMMARY

ACTS is characterized by rapid onset of median neuropathy caused by sudden increases in carpal tunnel pressures, which leads to ischemia of the median nerve. The most common cause is traumatic injury, although atraumatic sources should also be recognized. Patients generally lose two-point discrimination and may have elevated compartment pressure on measurement. Prompt recognition and surgical decompression are imperative to spare median nerve viability.

REFERENCES

1. Cranford CS, Ho JY, Kalainov DM, et al. Carpal tunnel syndrome. J Am Acad Orthop Surg 2007;15:537–48.
2. Michelsen H, Posner MA. Medical history of carpal tunnel syndrome. Hand Clin 2002;18:257–68.
3. Schnetzler KA. Acute carpal tunnel syndrome. J Am Acad Orthop Surg 2008;16(5):276–82 Review.
4. Szabo RM. Acute carpal tunnel syndrome. Hand Clin 1998;14:419–29.

5. Mack GR, McPherson SA, Lutz RB. Acute median neuropathy after wrist trauma: the role of emergent carpal tunnel release. Clin Orthop Relat Res 1994; 300:141–6, 1124.

6. Adamson JE, Srouji SJ, Horton CE, et al. The acute carpal tunnel syndrome. Plast Reconstr Surg 1971; 47:332–6.

7. Bauman TD, Gelberman RH, Mubarak SJ, et al. The acute carpal tunnel syndrome. Clin Orthop 1981; 156:151–6.

8. Cobb T, Dalley B, Posteraro R, et al. Anatomy of the flexor retinaculum. J Hand Surg 1993;18:91–9.

9. Rotman MB, Donovan JP. Practical anatomy of the carpal tunnel. Hand Clin 2002;18:219–30. J Neurol Neurosurg Psychiatry 1980;43:690–8.

10. Kozin S. The anatomy of the recurrent branch of the median nerve. J Hand Surg 1998;23:852–8.

11. Diao E, Shao F, Liebenberg E, et al. Carpal tunnel pressure alters median nerve function in a dose-dependent manner: a rabbit model for carpal tunnel syndrome. J Orthop Res 2005;23:218–23.

12. Ford DJ, Ali MS. Acute carpal tunnel syndrome: complications of delayed decompression. J Bone Joint Surg Br 1986;68:758–9.

13. Paget J. The first description of carpal tunnel syndrome. J Hand Surg Eur Vol 2007;32(2):195–7 [Epub 2007 Feb 12].

14. Frykman G. Fracture of the distal radius including sequelae-shoulder-hand-finger syndrome, disturbance in the distal radio-ulnar joint and impairment of nerve function. A clinical and experimental study. Acta Orthop Scand 1967;(Suppl 108):3.

15. Lewis MH. Median nerve decompression after Colles's fracture. J Bone Joint Surg Br 1978;60-B(2): 195–6.

16. Dyer G, Lozano-Calderon S, Gannon C, et al. Predictors of acute carpal tunnel syndrome associated with fracture of the distal radius. J Hand Surg Am 2008;33(8):1309–13.

17. Figus A, Iwuagwu FC, Elliot D. Subacute nerve compressions after trauma and surgery of the hand. Plast Reconstr Surg 2007;120(3):705–12.

18. Black PR, Flowers MJ, Saleh M. Acute carpal tunnel syndrome as a complication of oral anticoagulant therapy. J Hand Surg Br 1997;22:50–1.

19. Rahimtoola ZO, van Baal SG. Two cases of acute carpal tunnel syndrome in classic haemophilia. Scand J Plast Reconstr Surg Hand Surg 2002;36: 186–8.

20. Parthenis DG, Karagkevrekis CB, Waldram MA. von Willebrand's disease presenting as acute carpal tunnel syndrome. J Hand Surg Br 1998; 23:114.

21. Mahmud T. Bilateral acute carpal tunnel syndrome after combined pancreatic and renal transplant. Scand J Plast Reconstr Surg Hand Surg 2009; 43(3):174–6.

22. Ling SK, Cheng SC, Yen CH. Stonefish envenomation with acute carpal tunnel syndrome. Hong Kong Med J 2009;15(6):471–3.

23. Balakrishnan C, Mussman JL, Balakrishnan A, et al. Acute carpal tunnel syndrome from burns of the hand and wrist. Can J Plast Surg 2009;17(4):e33–4.

24. Gaur SC, Kulshreshtha K, Swarup S. Acute carpal tunnel syndrome in Hansen's disease. J Hand Surg Br 1994;19(3):286–7.

25. Gallagher B, Khalifa M, Van Heerden P, et al. Acute carpal tunnel syndrome due to filarial infection. Pathol Res Pract 2002;198(1):65–7.

26. Flynn JM, Bischoff R, Gelberman RH. Median nerve compression at the wrist due to intracarpal canal sepsis. J Hand Surg Am 1995;20(5):864–7.

27. Samii K, Cassinotti P, de Freudenreich J, et al. Acute bilateral carpal tunnel syndrome associated with human parvovirus B19 infection. Clin Infect Dis 1996;22(1):162–4.

28. El Hajj II, Harb MI, Sawaya RA. Acute progressive bilateral carpal tunnel syndrome after upper respiratory tract infection. South Med J 2005;98(11):1149–51.

29. Gerardi JA, Mack GR, Lutz RB. Acute carpal tunnel syndrome secondary to septic arthritis of the wrist. J Am Osteopath Assoc 1989;89(7):933–4.

30. Nourissat G, Fournier E, Werther JR, et al. Acute carpal tunnel syndrome secondary to pyogenic tenosynovitis. J Hand Surg Br 2006;31(6):687–8 [Epub 2006 Jul 25].

31. Chiu KY, Ng WF, Wong WB, et al. Acute carpal tunnel syndrome caused by pseudogout. J Hand Surg Am 1992;17(2):299–302.

32. Pai CH, Tseng CH. Acute carpal tunnel syndrome caused by tophaceous gout. J Hand Surg Am 1993;18(4):667–9.

33. McClain EJ, Wissinger HA. The acute carpal tunnel syndrome: nine case reports. J Trauma 1976;16(1): 75–8.

34. Rose RE. Acute carpal tunnel syndrome secondary to thrombosis of a persistent median artery. West Indian Med J 1995;44:32–3.

35. Dickinson JC, Kleinert JM. Acute carpal tunnel syndrome caused by a calcified median artery: a case report. J Bone Joint Surg Am 1991;73:610–1.

36. Faithfull DK, Wallace RF. Traumatic rupture of median artery: an unusual cause for acute median nerve compression. J Hand Surg Br 1987;12:233–5.

37. Wright C, MacFarlane I. Aneurysm of the median artery causing carpal tunnel syndrome. Aust N Z J Surg 1994;64:66–7.

38. Ametewee K, Harris A, Samuel M. Acute carpal tunnel syndrome produced by anomalous flexor digitorum superficialis indicis muscle. J Hand Surg Br 1985;10:83–4.

39. Jones DG, Savage R, Highton J. Synovitis induced by alendronic acid can present as acute carpal tunnel syndrome. BMJ 2005;330(7482):74.

40. Lundborg G, Gelberman RH, Minteer-Convery M, et al. Median nerve compression in the carpal tunnel: functional response to experimentally induced controlled pressure. J Hand Surg Am 1982; 7:252–9.

41. Szabo RM, Gelberman RH, Williamson RV, et al. Effects of increased systemic blood pressure on the tissue fluid pressure threshold of peripheral nerve. J Orthop Res 1983;1:172–8.

42. Lundborg G. Ischemic nerve injury. Experimental studies on intraneural microvascular pathophysiology and nerve function in a limb subjected to temporary circulatory arrest. Scand J Plast Reconstr Surg Suppl 1970;6:3–113.

Ulnar Tunnel Syndrome

Abdo Bachoura, MD[a], Sidney M. Jacoby, MD[a,b],*

KEYWORDS

- Ulnar nerve • Ulnar tunnel syndrome • Guyon's canal • Compressive neuropathy • Wrist • Hand

KEY POINTS

- A zone I compression elicits motor and sensory signs and symptoms, a zone II compression results in isolated motor deficits, and a zone III compression causes purely sensory deficits.
- In select cases, conservative treatment such as activity modification may be helpful, but often, surgical exploration of the ulnar tunnel with subsequent ulnar nerve decompression is indicated.
- The anatomy of the ulnar tunnel is complex, but numerous anatomic studies have described the tunnel in significant detail. Because organic lesions are often implicated in the cause, surgical exploration and decompression of the ulnar tunnel represent a common treatment modality.

INTRODUCTION

Ulnar tunnel syndrome (UTS) is broadly defined as a compressive neuropathy of the ulnar nerve at the level of the wrist. The term "ulnar tunnel syndrome" was coined by DuPont and colleagues[1] in 1965 to describe the condition of 4 patients with acquired ulnar neuritis. The ulnar tunnel proper, also known as "Guyon's canal," is one potential but not exclusive site of ulnar nerve compression at the wrist. The eponym comes from Guyon's description in 1861 of a space at the base of the hypothenar eminence at which the ulnar nerve bifurcates and that is vulnerable to compression from surrounding structures.[2,3] Numerous factors may precipitate the onset of UTS, including space-occupying lesions, vascular lesions, and repetitive trauma. Patient presentation depends on the anatomic zone of ulnar nerve compression and therefore may be purely motor, purely sensory, or a combination of both. In select cases, conservative treatment such as activity modification may be helpful, but often, surgical exploration of the ulnar tunnel with subsequent ulnar nerve decompression is indicated.

ANATOMY

As with all nerve-related disease, a thorough understanding of anatomy and potential sites of compression is critical. The ulnar nerve emerges from the medial cord (C8–T1) of the brachial plexus and passes through the axilla into the anterior compartment of the arm, before piercing the intermuscular septum and traveling in the posterior compartment medially. It then courses superficially and passes posterior to the medial epicondyle, into the anatomic cubital tunnel. The nerve then continues deep along the flexor digitorum profundus in the forearm. Before its entrance to the ulnar tunnel, approximately 3.4 cm proximal to the ulnar styloid, the ulnar nerve gives off the dorsal cutaneous branch, which innervates the ulnar and dorsal side of the hand.[4] The main nerve resurfaces at the level of the wrist where it passes through the ulnar tunnel, which is a fibro-osseous structure. The anatomy of the tunnel is complex, and variations in the nomenclature and structures surrounding the tunnel have previously been a source of confusion and misinterpretation.[5,6] For example, the terms *pisohamate tunnel*,[5,6] *pisohamate hiatus*,[6–8] and *pisohamate arcade*[6] have been used variably and interchangeably to describe the ulnar tunnel in part or whole. The entrance of the tunnel is triangular and begins at the proximal edge of the palmar carpal ligament. It extends distally to the fibrous arch of the hypothenar muscles at the level of the hook of the hamate and is approximately 40 to 45 mm in length. The

Disclosure: None of the authors have any financial conflicts of interest to declare.

a The Philadelphia Hand Center, Suite G114, 834 Chestnut Street, Philadelphia, PA 19107, USA; b Department of Orthopaedic Surgery, Thomas Jefferson University Hospital, 1015 Walnut Street, Philadelphia, PA 19107, USA
* Corresponding author. 700 South Henderson Road, Suite 200, King of Prussia, PA 19406.
E-mail address: smjacoby@handcenters.com

Orthop Clin N Am 43 (2012) 467–474
http://dx.doi.org/10.1016/j.ocl.2012.07.016
0030-5898/12/$ – see front matter © 2012 Elsevier Inc. All rights reserved.

boundaries of the tunnel vary along its length.[3,6] Generally, the roof of the canal consists of the palmar carpal ligament, palmaris brevis, and hypothenar connective tissue. The floor of the canal consists of the transverse carpal ligament, pisohamate ligament, pisometacarpal ligament, and the tendons of the flexor digitorum profundus and opponens digiti minimi. The medial wall of the canal is formed by the pisiform, the abductor digiti minimi, and the tendon of the flexor carpi ulnaris. The lateral wall is formed by the hook of the hamate, the transverse carpal ligament, and the flexor tendons.[3,9,10]

Within the boundaries of the canal lie the ulnar nerve, ulnar artery, accompanying veins, and connective fatty tissue.[6] The ulnar nerve lies slightly deep and ulnar to the ulnar artery. During its course in Guyon's canal, the ulnar nerve bifurcates into a superficial and a deep branch approximately 6 mm distal to the distal pole of the pisiform.[6] The superficial branch innervates the palmaris brevis and provides the sensory fibers over the hypothenar eminence and small and ring fingers. The motor branch of the nerve exits deep in the canal and courses around the ulnar edge of the hamulus and then runs radially between the abductor digiti minimi and flexor digit minimi and dorsal to the flexor tendons of the small finger (**Fig. 1**).[6,11]

Compression of the ulnar nerve at the wrist is not limited to the confines of the ulnar tunnel. Shea and McClain and, later, Gross and Gelberman studied the relationship between the symptoms of ulnar neuropathy and the anatomic location of nerve compression about the wrist.[3,11] They classified compressive ulnar neuropathy at the wrist into 3 types (**Fig. 2**). Type I syndrome,[11] or a zone I[3] compression, occurs as a result of nerve compression proximal to or within Guyon's canal, before any nerve bifurcation, and manifests as motor weakness of all the ulnar innervated intrinsic muscles and sensory deficits over the hypothenar eminence and the small and ring digits. Type II syndrome, or a zone II compression, manifests exclusively as motor weakness of the hand. The sensory branch is spared and therefore sensation along the ulnar nerve distribution remains intact. Compression of the deep ulnar branch may occur as it exits Guyon's canal at the level of the hamulus. Type III syndrome, or a zone III compression, occurs secondary to compression of the superficial sensory branch of the ulnar nerve and manifests as isolated sensory loss.

COMMON PATHWAY OF COMPRESSIVE PERIPHERAL NEUROPATHIES

The details of nerve degeneration and regeneration as a result of compression loading have been studied extensively over the past few decades and have yielded a tremendous amount of information regarding the pathophysiology of nerve compression.[12–19] In general, these studies have demonstrated that nerve injury correlates to both the degree and duration of compression, with both mechanical and ischemic factors contributing to neurologic dysfunction.[20] Situations such as trauma or sustained compression will induce the accumulation of edema into the endoneurial space of the nerve trunk.[21] Because of the diffusion barrier created by the perineurium and the lack of lymphatic vessels in the endoneurial space, the fluid may not easily escape. The result is an increase in endoneurial fluid pressure and encroachment of the normal endoneurial microcirculation. A study by Lundborg and colleagues showed that after 2 to 8 hours of experimental compression-induced ischemia (80 mm Hg) in nerves of animals, the endoneurial fluid pressure may increase rapidly and persist for 24 hours or longer.[22] Another example of metabolic conduction block is the sensory loss and motor paralysis that can occur after deflating the tourniquet around the upper arm. This type of metabolic block, caused by local arrest of intraneural microcirculation, is immediately reversible when the compression is removed. With extended compression, however, edema within the fascicles can result in increased endoneurial pressure, which could compromise endoneurial capillary flow for hours or days, potentially permanently affecting function of the nerve.[23]

CAUSES

No reports have specifically addressed the incidence and prevalence of UTS in the widespread population. It is generally accepted that the incidence of UTS is much less than that of either carpal tunnel syndrome (CTS) or cubital tunnel syndrome. Numerous factors may cause UTS, and in fact, a large proportion of the literature on UTS is dedicated to case reports that describe the various causes of the disease.[24–38] Shea and colleagues[11] reported that the mass effect of ganglion cysts and then occupational neuritis were the 2 leading causes of UTS. During the past several decades, however, reports on isolated ulnar neuropathy secondary to occupational activities have been scarce.[39] Other causes include benign lesions, hook of hamate fractures, ulnar artery pathologic conditions or aberrancy, deviant hypothenar muscles, and crystal deposition disease. Chronic, repetitive trauma or compression over the hypothenar eminence has also been implicated as a cause of UTS[40] and is not uncommon in long-distance cyclists.[41,42] Idiopathic disease has also been reported.[37] Several studies have reported a strong

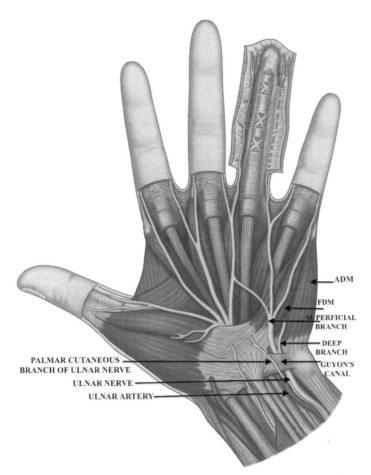

Fig. 1. Superficial structures of the palm and wrist. The superficial and deep branches of the ulnar nerve are indicated. ADM, abductor digiti minimi; FDM, flexor digiti minimi. (*From* Standring S. Gray's anatomy: the anatomical basis of clinical practice. 40th edition. New York: Churchill Livingstone; 2008. p. 891; with permission.)

association between the presentation of CTS and UTS,[1,43–46] whereas others have disputed this relationship.[47,48] The carpal and ulnar tunnels lie adjacent to each other. Although the transverse carpal ligament constitutes the roof of the carpal tunnel, it also constitutes the floor of the ulnar tunnel. Pressure changes within the carpal tunnel are transmitted to the ulnar tunnel, and vice versa. A relevant clinical correlate demonstrates this fact: to completely decompress the motor branch of the ulnar nerve, the transverse carpal ligament needs to be sectioned distally beyond the hook of the hamate, as the motor branch runs on the floor of the carpal tunnel. Silver and colleagues[46] reported a series of 59 hands with CTS and found concurrent ulnar sensory deficiencies in 34% of cases. After carpal tunnel release only, they found that 94% of their patients had improvements in ulnar nerve sensation according to the Semmes-Weinstein test. Ablove and colleagues[45] measured the pressure changes in the carpal tunnel and the

ulnar tunnel before and after endoscopic and open carpal tunnel release. Following the release, they found that pressure dropped significantly in both anatomic tunnels. They also suggested that carpal tunnel release alone could be used to successfully treat patients with concurrent disease. The association between CTS and UTS has been debated, but the trends in evidence seem to favor a true association between the two syndromes.

In sum, with regard to the cause of UTS, it seems that most cases are secondary to impingement of an organic lesion on a segment of the ulnar nerve. This contrasts with ulnar neuropathy at the elbow (cubital tunnel syndrome) or CTS, in which the most common causes are believed to be idiopathic.

HISTORY AND PHYSICAL EXAMINATION

A complete patient history includes information on cervical and any other peripheral joint pain (particularly elbow pain or trauma), the duration and

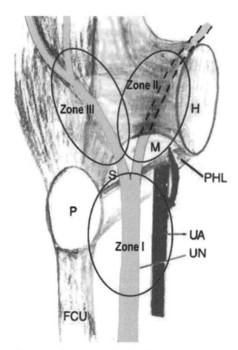

Fig. 2. Surgical anatomy in the Guyon canal and the 3 zones of injury as described by Gross and Gelberman. FCU, flexor carpi ulnaris; H, hamate; M, motor branch; P, pisiform; PHL, pisohamate ligament; S, sensory branch; UA, ulnar artery; UN, ulnar nerve. (*From* Kokkalis ZT, Efstathopoulos DG, Papanastassiou ID, et al. Ulnar nerve injuries in guyon canal: a report of 32 cases. Microsurgery 2012;32(4):296–302, with permission; and data from Gross MS, Gelberman RH. The anatomy of the distal ulnar tunnel. Clin Orthop Relat Res 1985;196:238–47.)

progress of symptoms, aggravating and relieving scenarios, and the common occupational or leisure activities. Patients with a history of club or racquet playing have been reported to suffer hamate fractures during instrument use,[49,50] whereas long-distance cyclers may acquire ulnar nerve compression as a result of prolonged grasping of the bicycle's handlebars and direct pressure on the wrist.[41,42] Manual labor that requires constant hammering or repetitive traumatic activities may damage the ulnar artery and perhaps the ulnar nerve as well, a condition often referred to as "hypothenar hammer syndrome."[40]

Ideally, the physical examination should rule out more proximal sites of nerve entrapment, and if possible, the examiner should be able to localize the zone of compression within the wrist. As a result, a thorough examination of the cervical spine and elbow is recommended. CTS should also be ruled out because of the likelihood of concurrent presentation. Careful observation for any gross masses over the dorsal or volar wrist is an important initial step. Hypothenar or interossei

wasting, clawing, or the inability to cross fingers may be observed in cases with motor branch involvement (**Fig. 3**).[1,28,38,51] Palpation may help in identifying the type and location of a lesion. Point tenderness over the hook of the hamate would place a hamulus fracture high in the differential diagnosis, whereas the hardness and consistency of any overt lesion may provide clues about the nature of the lesion. Vascular examination of the wrist is useful because UTS associated with ulnar artery pathology has been reported frequently.[26–28,34,37] Doppler examination for bruits or thrills over the ulnar artery may indicate pseudoaneurysmal dilation, and the Allen test may be useful to determine patency of the ulnar artery. Provocative tests such as the Tinel or Phalen test are often performed as part of the examination, but their usefulness has not been fully established. In 31 patients with type 1 disease (compression of both motor and sensory components of the ulnar nerve), Grundberg reported that 92% of his patients had a positive Phalen test, whereas the Tinel sign elicited paresthesias in only 44% of patients.[52] Objective tests that examine sensation, such as the Semmes-Weinstein monofilament test and 2-point static discrimination, can provide useful information about the location and magnitude of the disease and can provide baseline information. Similarly, comparing side-to-side grip strength and pinch strength can provide useful objective data to determine the initial status and gauge the progress of the intrinsic hand muscles.

DIAGNOSTIC TESTS

Imaging studies are useful for confirming a suspected diagnosis or when the cause is not entirely clear. If a hamulus fracture is suspected, a carpal view or hamate hook view radiograph or a computed tomography scan can provide useful information. Magnetic resonance imaging is frequently used

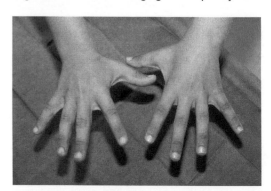

Fig. 3. First dorsal interosseous muscle wasting in the left hand. (*Courtesy of* Dr D.G. Efstathopoulos, KAT Accident Hospital, and Dr Z.T. Kokkalis, Attikon University Hospital, Athens, Greece.)

and is a suitable tool for localizing and diagnosing soft tissue masses, aberrant muscle, and vascular lesions, and it provides useful information for preoperative planning.[28,33,53,54] The use of ultrasound in UTS has not been fully investigated, but Harvie and colleagues[55] screened 58 asymptomatic volunteers to determine the prevalence and morphology of anomalous muscles within the ulnar and found that 47% of volunteers had anomalous variants of abductor digiti mini. It was not clear, however, how anomalous muscles were defined. Ultrasound has the advantages of being a noninvasive, safe, cost-effective tool that can aid in diagnosis,[35] and in select cases it may aid in ganglion aspiration.[56] Arteriography is appropriate when an ulnar artery pathologic condition is suspected.

Electrodiagnostic studies such as electromyography and nerve conduction studies are often used as confirmatory studies after positive motor tests and positive sensory findings to establish a diagnosis of nerve compression. Although not an adequate substitute for a thorough and detailed physical examination, quality electrodiagnostic studies can complement the clinical findings by localizing the lesion and predicting the likelihood of neural regeneration and recovery. Concerns include the highly operator-dependent nature of the tests and the confounding effect of systemic disease–related and age-related changes to expected values. Nerve conduction testing cannot objectively evaluate pain and paresthesias because these sensations are transmitted by unmyelinated fibers that are left untested in the setting of a study, which assesses large myelinated nerve tracts.

CONSERVATIVE TREATMENT

Nonoperative treatment is usually initiated in mild cases or when a specific structural abnormality has not been identified. Little evidence exists regarding the effectiveness of conservative treatment. Protective splinting and anti-inflammatory medications may be appropriate in mild cases and in the event of concurrent CTS and UTS.[1] Activity modification has been shown to be an effective intervention when the cause of UTS is related to repetitive compression or trauma.[35,39,41] Ganglion aspiration alone has been performed to successfully treat UTS.[56] Little or no evidence exists regarding the role of steroid injections into Guyon's canal for idiopathic cases.

SURGERY

If an organic compressive lesion is causing signs and symptoms or if conservative treatment has failed, the patient should be offered surgery. Surgical exploration, removal of any space-

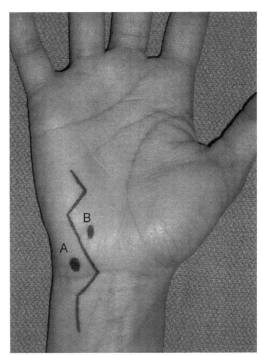

Fig. 4. Outline of a standard approach for decompression of the ulnar tunnel. The pisiform is labelled A, while the hook of the hamate is labelled B. (*Courtesy of* A.M. Ilyas.)

occupying lesion, and decompression of the ulnar tunnel form the standard surgical treatment.

Under either general, regional, or local anesthesia and tourniquet control, the patient's hand is placed in the supine position. It is our preference to perform this procedure under either general or regional anesthesia to avoid obscuring landmarks with local anesthetic administration; however, it certainly acceptable to use local anesthesia. An appropriate length incision is made longitudinally parallel to the thenar crease between

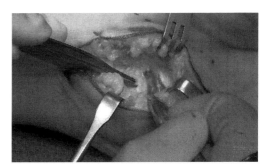

Fig. 5. Demonstration of the fibrous archlike origin of the hypothenar muscles. The hook of the hamate is ink-marked. The deep motor branch of the ulnar nerve courses deep to the fibrous arch. (*From* Washington University School of Medicine in St Louis. Peripheral nerve surgery: a resource for surgeons. Available at: nervesurgery.wustl.edu.)

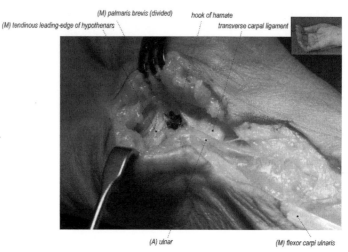

(M) palmaris brevis (divided)   *hook of hamate*
(M) tendinous leading-edge of hypothenars   *transverse carpal ligament*

(A) ulnar   *(M) flexor carpi ulnaris*

Fig. 6. Demonstration of the leading edge of the hypothenar muscles. (*From* Washington University School of Medicine in St Louis. Peripheral nerve surgery: a resource for surgeons. Available at: nervesurgery.wustl.edu.)

the hamulus and pisiform and extended proximally approximately 3 to 4 cm beyond the distal wrist crease (**Fig. 4**). The palmaris brevis is incised proximally. Farther distally along the incision, some patients may exhibit an ulnar palmar cutaneous branch of large caliber. It is preferable to preserve this branch to limit postoperative paresthesias. Moving deep to the incision proximally, the thick antebrachial fascia over the proximal wrist is released to decompress the ulnar nerve in zone I. Once the roof of Guyon's canal is released, the contents of the canal, particularly the ulnar artery and ulnar nerve before bifurcation, should be visible and accessible. The neurovascular bundle is gently moved medially and the hook of the hamate is identified. The fibrous, archlike origin of the hypothenar muscles should become evident coming off the hook of hamate (**Figs. 5 and 6**). Beneath the arch lies the deep motor branch of the ulnar nerve. The tendinous hypothenar muscle origin is carefully released close to the hook to further decompress the distal end the tunnel. The superficial sensory branch of the ulnar nerve courses superficial to the fibrous arch or the hypothenar muscles. Throughout the procedure, the ulnar artery should be carefully inspected to rule out any overt vascular pathologic condition. After completion of the decompression, the tourniquet is deflated and adequate hemostasis is ensured. The wound is closed and a bulky dressing or plaster splint is applied. Sutures are frequently removed at 10 to 14 days postoperatively.

SUMMARY

The approach to the diagnosis and treatment of UTS has changed little during the past several decades. UTS is less common than either CTS or cubital tunnel syndrome, and in a high proportion of cases, the cause can be localized to a compressive space-occupying lesion or repetitive trauma. The anatomy of the ulnar tunnel is complex, but numerous anatomic studies have described the tunnel in significant detail. Because organic lesions are often implicated in the cause, surgical exploration and decompression of the ulnar tunnel is a common treatment modality. Reported surgical results have yielded good results, although at this time, case series and comparative studies are uncommon, perhaps as a result of both the infrequency and heterogeneity of the causes.

REFERENCES

1. Dupont C, Cloutier GE, Prevost Y, et al. Ulnar-tunnel syndrome at the wrist. A report of four cases ulnar-nerve compression at the wrist. J Bone Joint Surg Am 1965;47:757–61.
2. Guyon F. Note sur une disposition anatomique propre á la face anté rieure de la region du poignet et non encore dé crite par le docteur. Bulletins de la Societe Anatomique de Paris Second Series 1861;6: 184 [in French].
3. Gross MS, Gelberman RH. The anatomy of the distal ulnar tunnel. Clin Orthop Relat Res 1985;196:238–47.
4. Goto A, Kunihiro O, Murase T, et al. The dorsal cutaneous branch of the ulnar nerve: an anatomical study. Hand Surg 2010;15(3):165–8.
5. Bozkurt MC. Anatomy of the ulnar tunnel and the influence of wrist motion on its morphology. J Hand Surg Am 2010;35:1719 [author reply: 1719–20].
6. Ombaba J, Kuo M, Rayan G. Anatomy of the ulnar tunnel and the influence of wrist motion on its morphology. J Hand Surg Am 2010;35(10):760–8.

7. Uriburu IJ, Morchio FJ, Marin JC. Compression syndrome of the deep motor branch of the ulnar nerve. (Piso-Hamate Hiatus syndrome). J Bone Joint Surg Am 1976;58(1):145–7.

8. Bozkurt MC, Tagil SM, Ozcakar L, et al. Anatomical variations as potential risk factors for ulnar tunnel syndrome: a cadaveric study. Clin Anat 2005; 18(4):274–80.

9. Pierre-Jerome C, Moncayo V, Terk MR. The Guyon's canal in perspective: 3-T MRI assessment of the normal anatomy, the anatomical variations and the Guyon's canal syndrome. Surg Radiol Anat 2011; 33(10):897–903.

10. Zeiss J, Jakab E, Khimji T, et al. The ulnar tunnel at the wrist (Guyon's canal): normal MR anatomy and variants. AJR Am J Roentgenol 1992;158(5): 1081–5.

11. Shea JD, McClain EJ. Ulnar-nerve compression syndromes at and below the wrist. J Bone Joint Surg Am 1969;51(6):1095–103.

12. Dellon AL, Mackinnon SE. Chronic nerve compression model for the double crush hypothesis. Ann Plast Surg 1991;26(3):259–64.

13. Gelberman RH, Szabo RM, Williamson RV, et al. Sensibility testing in peripheral-nerve compression syndromes. An experimental study in humans. J Bone Joint Surg Am 1983;65(5):632–8.

14. Mackinnon SE, Dellon AL. Evaluation of microsurgical internal neurolysis in a primate median nerve model of chronic nerve compression. J Hand Surg Am 1988;13(3):345–51.

15. Mackinnon SE, Dellon AL, Hudson AR, et al. A primate model for chronic nerve compression. J Reconstr Microsurg 1985;1(3):185–95.

16. Mackinnon SE, Dellon AL, Hudson AR, et al. Chronic human nerve compression: a histological assessment. Neuropathol Appl Neurobiol 1986;12(6):547–65.

17. O'Brien JP, Mackinnon SE, MacLean AR, et al. A model of chronic nerve compression in the rat. Ann Plast Surg 1987;19(5):430–5.

18. Rempel D, Dahlin L, Lundborg G. Pathophysiology of nerve compression syndromes: response of peripheral nerves to loading. J Bone Joint Surg Am 1999;81(11):1600–10.

19. Szabo RM, Gelberman RH, Williamson RV, et al. Vibratory sensory testing in acute peripheral nerve compression. J Hand Surg Am 1984;9A(1):104–9.

20. Mackinnon SE. Pathophysiology of nerve compression. Hand Clin 2002;18(2):231–41.

21. Lundborg G. Structure and function of the intraneural microvessels as related to trauma, edema formation, and nerve function. J Bone Joint Surg Am 1975; 57(7):938–48.

22. Lundborg G, Myers R, Powell H. Nerve compression injury and increased endoneurial fluid pressure: a "miniature compartment syndrome." J Neurol Neurosurg Psychiatry 1983;46(12):1119–24.

23. Lundborg G, Dahlin LB. Anatomy, function, and pathophysiology of peripheral nerves and nerve compression. Hand Clin 1996;12(2):185–93.

24. Chammas M, Meyer zu Reckendorf G, Allieu Y. Compression of the ulnar nerve in Guyon's canal by pseudotumoral calcinosis in systemic scleroderma. J Hand Surg Br 1995;20(6):794–6.

25. Dell PC. Compression of the ulnar nerve at the wrist secondary to a rheumatoid synovial cyst: case report and review of the literature. J Hand Surg Am 1979;4(5):468–73.

26. Jose RM, Bragg T, Srivastava S. Ulnar nerve compression in Guyon's canal in the presence of a tortuous ulnar artery. J Hand Surg Br 2006;31(2):200–2.

27. Kalisman M, Laborde K, Wolff TW. Ulnar nerve compression secondary to ulnar artery false aneurysm at the Guyon's canal. J Hand Surg Am 1982; 7(2):137–9.

28. Koch H, Haas F, Pierer G. Ulnar nerve compression in Guyon's canal due to a haemangioma of the ulnar artery. J Hand Surg Br 1998;23(2):242–4.

29. Zahrawi F. Acute compression ulnar neuropathy at Guyon's canal resulting from lipoma. J Hand Surg Am 1984;9(2):238–9.

30. Nakamichi K, Tachibana S, Kitajima I. Ultrasonography in the diagnosis of ulnar tunnel syndrome caused by an occult ganglion. J Hand Surg Br 2000;25(5):503–4.

31. Stern PJ, Vice M. Compression of the deep branch of the ulnar nerve: a case report. J Hand Surg Am 1983;8(1):72–4.

32. Yamazaki H, Uchiyama S, Kato H. Median nerve and ulnar nerve palsy caused by calcium pyrophosphate dihydrate crystal deposition disease: case report. J Hand Surg Am 2008;33(8):1325–8.

33. Chen WA, Barnwell JC, Li Y, et al. An ulnar intraneural ganglion arising from the pisotriquetral joint: case report. J Hand Surg Am 2011;36(1):65–7.

34. Miyamoto W, Yamamoto S, Kii R, et al. Vascular leiomyoma resulting in ulnar neuropathy: case report. J Hand Surg Am 2008;33(10):1868–70.

35. Ginanneschi F, Filippou G, Milani P, et al. Ulnar nerve compression neuropathy at Guyon's canal caused by crutch walking: case report with ultrasonographic nerve imaging. Arch Phys Med Rehabil 2009;90(3): 522–4.

36. Budny PG, Regan PJ, Roberts AH. Localized nodular synovitis: a rare cause of ulnar nerve compression in Guyon's canal. J Hand Surg Am 1992;17(4):663–4.

37. Murata K, Shih JT, Tsai TM. Causes of ulnar tunnel syndrome: a retrospective study of 31 subjects. J Hand Surg Am 2003;28(4):647–51.

38. Thurman RT, Jindal P, Wolff TW. Ulnar nerve compression in Guyon's canal caused by calcinosis in scleroderma. J Hand Surg Am 1991;16(4):739–41.

39. Zambelis T, Karandreas N, Piperos P. Mononeuropathy of the deep motor palmar branch of the ulnar

nerve: report of two unusual cases. J Orthopaed Traumatol 2005;6(2):95–7.

40. Marie I, Herve F, Primard E, et al. Long-term follow-up of hypothenar hammer syndrome: a series of 47 patients. Medicine (Baltimore) 2007;86(6):334–43.

41. Patterson JM, Jaggars MM, Boyer MI. Ulnar and median nerve palsy in long-distance cyclists. A prospective study. Am J Sports Med 2003;31(4):585–9.

42. Akuthota V, Plastaras C, Lindberg K, et al. The effect of long-distance bicycling on ulnar and median nerves: an electrophysiologic evaluation of cyclist palsy. Am J Sports Med 2005;33(8):1224–30.

43. Kiylioglu N, Akyildiz UO, Ozkul A, et al. Carpal tunnel syndrome and ulnar neuropathy at the wrist: comorbid disease or not? J Clin Neurophysiol 2011;28(5):520–3.

44. Chiodo A, Chadd E. Ulnar neuropathy at or distal to the wrist: traumatic versus cumulative stress cases. Arch Phys Med Rehabil 2007;88(4):504–12.

45. Ablove RH, Moy OJ, Peimer CA, et al. Pressure changes in Guyon's canal after carpal tunnel release. J Hand Surg Br 1996;21(5):664–5.

46. Silver MA, Gelberman RH, Gellman H, et al. Carpal tunnel syndrome: associated abnormalities in ulnar nerve function and the effect of carpal tunnel release on these abnormalities. J Hand Surg Am 1985;10(5):710–3.

47. Moghtaderi A, Ghafarpoor M. The dilemma of ulnar nerve entrapment at wrist in carpal tunnel syndrome. Clin Neurol Neurosurg 2009;111(2):151–5.

48. Vahdatpour B, Raissi GR, Hollisaz MT. Study of the ulnar nerve compromise at the wrist of patients with carpal tunnel syndrome. Electromyogr Clin Neurophysiol 2007;47(3):183–6.

49. Futami T, Aoki H, Tsukamoto Y. Fractures of the hook of the hamate in athletes. 8 cases followed for 6 years. Acta Orthop Scand 1993;64(4):469–71.

50. Stark HH, Jobe FW, Boyes JH, et al. Fracture of the hook of the hamate in athletes. J Bone Joint Surg Am 1977;59(5):575–82.

51. Packer NP, Fisk GR. Compression of the distal ulnar nerve with clawing of the index finger. Hand 1982;14(1):38–40.

52. Grundberg AB. Ulnar tunnel syndrome. J Hand Surg Br 1984;9(1):72–4.

53. Subin GD, Mallon WJ, Urbaniak JR. Diagnosis of ganglion in Guyon's canal by magnetic resonance imaging. J Hand Surg Am 1989;14(4):640–3.

54. Ruocco MJ, Walsh JJ, Jackson JP. MR imaging of ulnar nerve entrapment secondary to an anomalous wrist muscle. Skeletal Radiol 1998;27(4):218–21.

55. Harvie P, Patel N, Ostlere SJ. Prevalence and epidemiological variation of anomalous muscles at guyon's canal. J Hand Surg Br 2004;29(1):26–9.

56. Nakamichi K, Tachibana S. Ganglion-associated ulnar tunnel syndrome treated by ultrasonographically assisted aspiration and splinting. J Hand Surg Br 2003;28(2):177–8.

Cubital Tunnel Syndrome

Leo T. Kroonen, MD

KEYWORDS

- Ulnar nerve • Cubital tunnel • Peripheral nerve • Compression syndrome • Nerve transposition
- Medial epicondylectomy

KEY POINTS

- Compression of the ulnar nerve at the elbow, or cubital tunnel syndrome, is the second most common peripheral nerve compression syndrome in the upper extremity.
- Surgical intervention is indicated when nonoperative treatment, including activity modification, does not relieve the symptoms.
- There is currently no consensus on the best surgical treatment of cubital tunnel syndrome.

INTRODUCTION

In 1878, Panas[1] provided the first description of ulnar neuropathy across the elbow in a patient who had sustained an elbow fracture as a child and developed a tardy ulnar nerve palsy. With subsequent descriptions throughout the early 1900s, investigators focused on specific origins of these symptoms related to trauma and osteoarthritis, often referring to the constellation of symptoms as a "friction neuritis" or "traumatic neuritis."[2]

It was not until 1949 that Magee and Phalen[3] described the first case of a spontaneous presentation of ulnar nerve symptoms across the elbow. They suggested the cubital tunnel as the origin of the symptoms.[3,4] Osborne[4] (1957) described a fibrous band bridging the 2 heads of the flexor carpi ulnaris (FCU) as a site of compression and was the first to recommend a release of the cubital tunnel and anterior transposition of the nerve.[5] One year later, Feindel and Stratford[5] compared this compressive neuropathy with carpal tunnel syndrome as "an area of focal constriction" and recommended simple decompression to relieve the symptoms.

Since the 1950s, the diagnosis of cubital tunnel syndrome has increased in prevalence to become the second most common compressive neuropathy in the upper extremity after carpal tunnel syndrome.[6,7] The purpose of this article is to review the relevant anatomy of ulnar neuropathy across the elbow, the proposed causes, and to review the relevant diagnostic maneuvers and treatment options to provide the reader with a logical approach to treating this common entity.

ANATOMY

An understanding of the anatomic course of the ulnar nerve is critical to understanding cubital tunnel syndrome and its differential diagnoses.

The Course of the Ulnar Nerve

The ulnar nerve proper travels the following course:

- Originates in the axilla from the medial cord of the brachial plexus, with contributions from the C8-T1 nerve roots

Disclosures: The views presented are those of the author and do not represent the official views of the US Government, the Department of Defense, or the Department of the Navy. The author has no financial disclosures directly related to this topic.
Hand & Microvascular Surgery, Department of Orthopedic Surgery, Naval Medical Center San Diego, 34800 Bob Wilson Drive, San Diego, CA 92134, USA
E-mail address: leo.kroonen@med.navy.mil

Orthop Clin N Am 43 (2012) 475–486
http://dx.doi.org/10.1016/j.ocl.2012.07.017
0030-5898/12/$ – see front matter Published by Elsevier Inc.

- Travels posterior to the medial intermuscular septum, anterior to the medial head of the triceps
- Through the cubital tunnel (defined later)
- Dives into the forearm between the 2 heads of the FCU
- Travels between the FCU and flexor digitorum profundus into the forearm
- Travels through Guyon canal at the wrist
  - Terminates in the hand as motor and sensory branches
    - Sensory: ulnar digital nerve to the ring finger, radial and ulnar digital nerves to the small finger
    - Motor: deep motor branch to the intrinsic muscles of the hand

Significant branches of the ulnar nerve during the dissection around the cubital tunnel include the following:

- The first branch off the ulnar nerve in most patients is a sensory branch to the elbow joint. It can be sacrificed without significant consequence.
- The next branch is a motor branch to the FCU.
  - Often times this branch is a tether to anterior transposition of the nerve and must be freed via neurolysis to a more proximal level to complete the transposition.

Sites of Compression of the Ulnar Nerve (Proximal to Distal)

Nerve fibers contributing to the ulnar nerve begin in the neck and travel all the way down to the fingertips of the ring and small fingers, sending branches out along the way (**Fig. 1**). Entrapment of these nerve fibers at any point along this path can cause symptoms. For the purpose of this article, only compression along the ulnar nerve from the brachium through the area of the cubital tunnel is discussed. The common sites of compression include the following:

- Arcade of Struthers (a fibrous band running from the medial head of the triceps to the medial intermuscular septum) located approximately 8 cm proximal to medial epicondyle
  - Arcade of Struthers present in 70% of patients[8]
  - Implicated primarily as a site of compression in the *transposed* nerve
- Medial intermuscular septum: also implicated primarily as a site of compression in the *transposed* nerve
- Medial epicondyle of the humerus
- Arcuate ligament of Osborne/cubital tunnel proper
  - Osborne ligament: the thickened fascia between ulnar and humeral heads of the flexor carpi ulnaris that creates the roof of the cubital tunnel
  - The floor of the cubital tunnel is formed by the medial collateral ligament of the elbow
- Anconeus epitrochlearis: anomalous muscle present in 1% to 30% of people that overlies the nerve and runs from its origin on the medial epicondyle to the olecranon (**Fig. 2**)[9]
- Fibrous bands within the FCU
- Aponeurosis at the proximal edge of the flexor digitorum sublimis

Extrinsic Blood Supply of the Ulnar Nerve

The extrinsic blood supply has been discussed as a potential concern in ulnar neuropathy (**Fig. 3**).

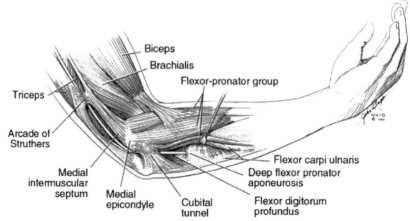

Fig. 1. Site of compression of the ulnar nerve at the elbow (By permission of Mayo Foundation for Medical Education and Research. All rights reserved.).

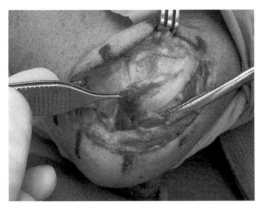

Fig. 2. Anconeus epitrochlearis: The ulnar nerve can be seen traversing through the anomalous muscle belly at the cubital tunnel.

Smith[10] (1966) reported that if the nerve was dissected over a distance of 6 to 8 cm, a portion of the nerve would be devascularized.[10,11] The ulnar nerve receives its blood supply from 3 main branches:

- Superior ulnar collateral artery
- Posterior ulnar recurrent artery
- Inferior ulnar collateral artery (variably present)[12]

Because the nerve has already been compromised in cases of ulnar neuropathy, efforts should be made to maintain as much of the extrinsic blood supply as possible when performing ulnar nerve surgery.

Surrounding Anatomic Dangers

In addition to the nerve itself, 2 main structures are at risk when performing ulnar nerve surgery:

- Posterior branches of the medial antebrachial cutaneous nerve are particularly at

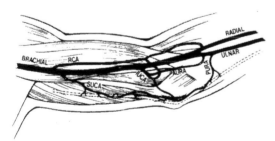

Fig. 3. Extrinsic blood supply to the ulnar nerve. IUCA, inferior ulnar collateral artery; PURA, posterior ulnar recurrent artery; SUCA, superior ulnar collateral artery. (*From* Prevel CD, Matloub HS, Ye Z, et al. The extrinsic blood supply of the ulnar nerve at the elbow: an anatomic study. J Hand Surg 1993;18A:433–38; with permission.)

risk in anterior transposition surgeries with longer incisions.
- ○ Sixty-one percent of patients have branches crossing approximately 1.8 cm proximal to the medial epicondyle.
- ○ One hundred percent of patients have branches crossing approximately 3.1 cm distal to the medial epicondyle.[13]
- The medial collateral ligament of the elbow forms the floor of the cubital tunnel and is at risk when performing a medial epicondylectomy.[2]

CAUSE

Most surgeons agree that there are 2 main factors that play a role in idiopathic ulnar neuropathy of the elbow: compression and traction.

- Feindel and Stratford[5] reported that the normally oval configuration of the cubital tunnel changes to a more slitlike shape with elbow flexion.
- Iba and colleagues[14] reported on intraoperative pressures in the cubital tunnel and found them to be elevated to an average of 105 mm Hg, compared with normal pressures reported in cadavers that were previously reported to be between 17 to 65 mm Hg.
- Other investigators have suggested that the course around the medial epicondyle creates increased tensile strain along the nerve as the elbow moves into flexion.
  - ○ Gelberman and colleagues[15] examined interstitial nerve pressures in the cubital tunnel and found that pressures were increased in elbow flexion even after release of the Osborne ligament.
  - ○ Hicks and Toby[16] found that performing a medial epicondylectomy and allowing anterior translation of the nerve was effective in decreasing strain in the nerve.

CLINICAL PRESENTATION
History

A detailed history and physical examination will usually reveal the diagnosis of cubital tunnel syndrome. Common presenting symptoms include the following:

- Vague discomfort localizing to the medial elbow
- Paresthesias or numbness in the ring and small fingers of the hand
- Weakness with grip and/or pinch strength
- Difficulty with opening jars or bottles

- Fatigue with repetitive tasks involving the hands
- Worsening of symptoms at night or with flexion of the elbow, such as when talking on the telephone

The categorization of symptoms has been described by McGowan[17] and modified by Dellon (**Box 1**).[18]

Physical Examination

- Observation alone can yield many findings in patients with cubital tunnel syndrome.
  - The carrying angle will give a clue as to whether there has been prior trauma that could increase the carrying angle and cause excess traction on the ulnar nerve.
  - Atrophy of the intrinsic muscles of the hand and, in particular, the first dorsal interosseous muscle is more common in severe ulnar neuropathy.
  - Clawing of the small and ring fingers is found in severe disease (Duchenne sign).
- The elbow range of motion should be assessed and will also suggest whether or not patients have underlying joint abnormalities, such as degenerative arthritis, which could be contributing to the symptoms.
- Sensory function should be assessed on both the radial and ulnar side of each digit to determine if there is altered sensibility in an anatomic pattern that corresponds to the ulnar nerve (ulnar side of ring finger and both radial and ulnar sides of small finger).
  - Light touch is useful as a quick screening test to determine if patients have gross subjective alteration in sensibility.
  - Monofilament testing/2-point discrimination (static) is useful for the evaluation of slow-adapting fibers.
  - Vibrometry/2-point discrimination (moving) is useful for the evaluation of quick-adapting fibers.

- Motor strength testing: Motor strength should be assessed in all of the major upper extremity muscle groups, with particular attention paid to the intrinsic muscles of the hand and the deep flexors to the ring and small fingers (**Fig. 4**). In addition, the following tests should be included in the examination:
  - Wartenberg sign (**Fig. 5**): Patients are unable to fully adduct the small finger and hold the finger slightly abducted and extended as the abductor digiti minimi is unopposed by the denervated palmar interosseous muscle.
  - Froment sign (**Fig. 6**): Patients are asked to perform a key (appositional) pinch. A positive test is indicated by the flexion of the interphalangeal joint of the thumb because patients attempt to compensate for weakness of the ulnar nerve innervated adductor pollicis by using the flexor pollicis longus (median nerve innervated).
- Provocative testing: Several physical examination maneuvers have been described to test the presence of ulnar neuropathy at the elbow. They include the following:
  - Tinel: This maneuver is performed by tapping over the course of the nerve with a finger. A positive test is elicited if tapping over the nerve reproduces paresthesias along the distribution of the ulnar nerve.
  - Elbow flexion-compression test: Patients are asked to hold their elbow in maximal flexion while the examiner holds pressure of the ulnar nerve at the cubital tunnel. A positive test reproduces paresthesias along the distribution of the ulnar nerve.
  - Scratch-collapse test (**Fig. 7**): With elbows at the side, patients forcibly externally rotate and abduct the forearms against resistance. The examiner then gently scratches along the course of the ulnar nerve at the elbow and then reapplies resistive force. A positive test is recorded if patients have a momentary loss in the ability to externally rotate against the examiner.[19]

ELECTRODIAGNOSTICS

In most cases, the history and physical examination alone will allow for the diagnosis of cubital tunnel syndrome. However, routine electrodiagnostic testing serves the following functions:

- Tests for nerve compression in other locations in addition to the cubital tunnel (ie, *double crush* phenomenon, with

Box 1
McGowan classification of ulnar nerve dysfunction
Grade I: Sensory neuropathy only
Grade II: Sensory and motor neuropathy, without muscle atrophy
Grade III: Sensory and motor neuropathy, muscle atrophy present

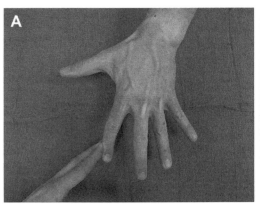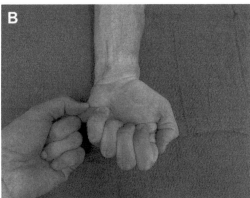

Fig. 4. Motor strength testing for ulnar neuropathy. (*A*) Testing the first dorsal interosseous muscle: Resistance is held against the fully abducted index finger. (*B*) Testing the deep flexor of the small finger: The patient is asked to make a fist around the examiner's finger, and resistance is applied against the flexed distal interphalangeal joint of the small finger.

compression in the cervical spine or more distally at Guyon canal)

- Can be useful for counseling patients regarding prognosis after surgery (Cases in which there are significant changes in the electromyogram (EMG) are less likely to completely resolve after surgery.)
- For cases in which the diagnosis is uncertain, whether because of a patient who is a poor historian or because of anatomic anomalies that can lead to atypical examination findings, such as the following:
  - Martin-Gruber communication: proximal forearm communication between the anterior interosseous nerve and the ulnar nerve (Deep finger flexors might not maintain their normal split innervation in this case.)
  - Riche-Cannieu anastomosis: anomalous communication in the hand between the deep motor branch of the ulnar nerve and the recurrent motor branch of the median nerve (In this case, the lumbrical might be median nerve innervated.[7])

- The diagnosis of cubital tunnel can still be made is patients who do not have electrodiagnostic abnormalities. When symptoms are caused by a subluxating nerve, the clinical symptoms might be present, but no slowing of conduction velocities is seen because there is no compression of the nerve.

Diagnostic Criteria for Cubital Tunnel Syndrome

A decrease in absolute conduction velocity to less than 50 m/s or a relative drop in conduction velocity of 10 m/s or more across a segment (usually the cubital tunnel). Inching studies are useful in positive tests to provide the surgeon with the site of maximal compression of the nerve.

DIFFERENTIAL DIAGNOSIS

- Cervical radiculopathy/brachial plexopathy
- Ulnar neuropathy at the wrist
- Medial epicondylitis

NONOPERATIVE TREATMENT

All patients presenting with mild symptoms of cubital tunnel syndrome should have a trial of nonsurgical treatment. In one study examining conservative treatment of cubital tunnel, 89.5% of patients demonstrated improvement in their symptoms at the 3-month follow-up.[20]

Activity Modification

Patients can be educated about positions to be avoided, particularly elbow flexion, such as when talking on the telephone, or positions in which the medial elbow is resting on a hard surface, such as elbows on arm rests when working on a computer.

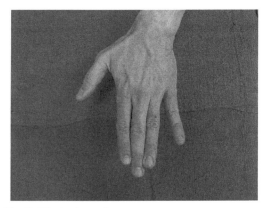

Fig. 5. Wartenberg sign.

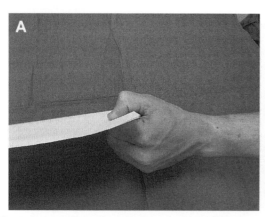
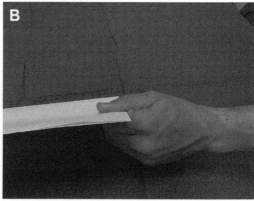

Fig. 6. Froment sign: The patient is asked to hold the paper between the thumb and index finger. (*A*) With the intact ulnar nerve, the patient is able to make use of the adductor pollicis. (*B*) When the ulnar nerve is deficient, the patient compensates for the denervated adductor by using the flexor pollicis longus (median nerve innervated).

Splinting

Nighttime flexion-blocking splints can be helpful to prevent patients from sleeping in deep elbow flexion.

Nerve Glides

Referral to occupational therapy for nerve-gliding exercises has been shown to be helpful in relieving symptoms of cubital tunnel syndrome in some studies.[20,21]

OPERATIVE TREATMENT

Surgical intervention is indicated when nonoperative treatment fails to provide adequate relief of symptoms. Several different procedures have

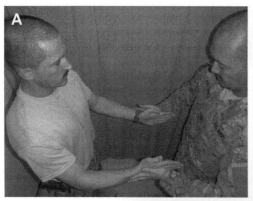
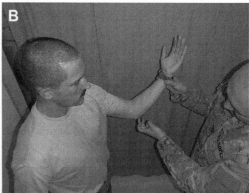
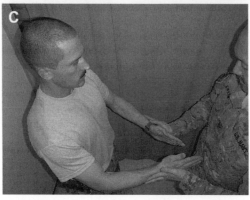

Fig. 7. MacKinnon's scratch collapse test: (*A*) The patient is asked to externally rotate the arms against resistance. (*B*) The examiner then scratches lightly over the course of the affected ulnar nerve. (*C*) In cases of cubital tunnel syndrome, the patient reflexively loses the ability to externally rotate the arm.

been described for the treatment of ulnar neuropathy at the elbow, but there is currently no consensus on the optimum treatment.

In Situ Decompression

The simplest technique for treating cubital tunnel is in situ decompression (**Fig. 8**). This procedure can be performed under local anesthesia (with or without sedation or general anesthesia if warranted in the particular patient).

- A 4-cm incision is made midway between the olecranon and medial epicondyle (see **Fig. 8**A).
- The ulnar nerve can usually be palpated proximal to the medial epicondyle and just posterior to the medial intermuscular septum. Tenotomy scissors can then be used to make a small opening in the sheath surrounding the nerve (see **Fig. 8**B). The author prefers to cheat this opening and the ensuing dissection slightly more posteriorly to leave a flap of tissue that can prevent nerve subluxation in mild cases (see **Fig. 8**C).
- Once the nerve is clearly identified, the dissection can be continued distally, opening the sheath over the ulnar nerve. A clear and easy plane can be found just superficial to the nerve, which allows dissection to continue easily around the epicondyle.
- In most cases, there is a thickening of the layer of tissue superficial to the nerve as

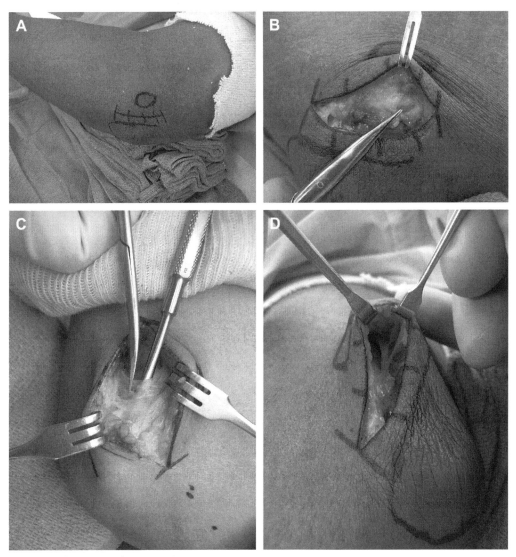

Fig. 8. In situ ulnar nerve decompression.

the turn is made around the medial epicondyle. This thickening is Osborne's Ligament (the beginning of the cubital tunnel proper).

- Dissection should proceed to completely open the cubital tunnel. This dissection will also include opening the superficial fascia of the FCU over a length of 2 to 3 cm.
- Special attention is then paid to the course of the nerve as it enters the FCU muscle. Often there are fascial bands deep to the superficial fascia that can cause constriction of the nerve. Any such bands should also be cut, thus ensuring that no bands are compressing the ulnar nerve within the FCU muscle.
- The literature is divided on whether or not to perform a more proximal release. Because it adds little time or difficulty to the case, the author routinely performs a proximal release of the nerve. By using a well-directed light and small retractors, the course of the nerve can be followed proximally, and blunt-tipped Metzenbaum scissors can be used to carefully slide along the nerve superficially to release the sheath around the nerve more proximally, including the arcade of Struthers, if present (see **Fig. 8D**).
- Once the nerve is completely released, the elbow should be taken through a full range of motion, paying special attention to the nerve's tendency toward subluxation. (If the nerve seems to move beyond the tip of the medial epicondyle with elbow flexion, then an anterior transposition or a medial epicondylectomy should be considered.)
- The skin is then closed per surgeon preference, and a soft dressing is placed.
- *Postoperative treatment*: Patients are allowed immediate elbow range of motion on the day of surgery. Activities can be progressed as tolerated and as the soft tissues allow.

Endoscopic Cubital Tunnel Release

First described in 1995 by Tsai, endoscopic techniques continue to emerge for performing ulnar nerve release at the elbow.[22–24]

- Watts and Bain[25] reported improved patient satisfaction with endoscopic release in a comparative analysis of endoscopic versus in situ release, but there were no statistically significant differences in objective outcomes.
- Various techniques have been described and involve the use of various pushing

devices to crease a space between the sheath around the nerve and the subcutaneous tissues. Then under endoscopic visualization, the sheath is opened over the nerve both proximally and distally in a similar fashion to an open in situ release.

- Incisions are typically reported to be 15 to 30 mm.
- A subluxating ulnar nerve on clinical examination is typically considered to be a contraindication to endoscopic release.

Medical Epicondylectomy

First described by King[26] in 1959, medial epicondylectomy is an attempt to eliminate the traction placed on the nerve as it courses around the epicondyle, especially in a flexed position. By performing a medial epicondylectomy, the roadblock for the ulnar nerve is removed, and the nerve is allowed to find it's own natural resting place in a more anterior position. Strain across the nerve is significantly decreased after a medial epicondylectomy compared with in situ release alone.[16] The technique is performed as follows:

- Medial epicondylectomy is a procedure performed in conjunction with an in situ decompression for cases in which the ulnar nerve subluxates over the medial epicondyle after release.
- After the nerve has been released, it is carefully protected by placing a Penrose drain around the nerve to gently retract it away from the epicondyle.
- The epicondyle itself is then longitudinally exposed subperiosteally. Once fully exposed, an osteotome is used to resect the epicondyle (**Fig. 9**).
- Once the desired amount of bone is resected, the soft tissues, including the periosteum, are repaired using a buried absorbable suture to prevent the nerve from lying over exposed bone.
- There is no consensus on what the ideal amount of bone is to remove.
  - In his original description of the procedure, King advocated the removal of the medial epicondyle to a level flush with the medial edge of the trochlea.
  - Heithoff[2] reported that after complete epicondylectomy, radiographic stress views did demonstrate medial instability and, thus, advocated preserving at least a portion of the fibers of the medial collateral ligament.

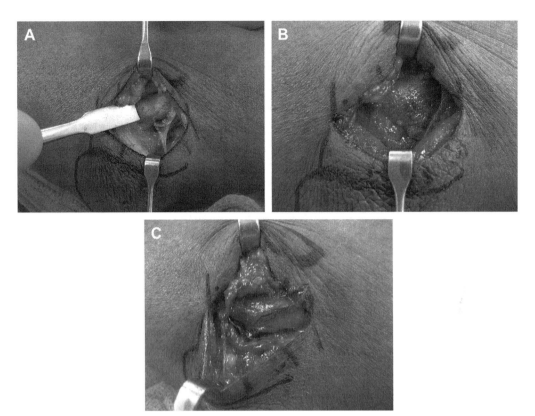

Fig. 9. Technique for medial epicondylectomy: (*A*) A small osteotome is used to resect 5 to 8 mm of epicondyle that has been subperiosteally exposed. (*B*) The cancellous bone is then exposed. A small amount of bone wax can be used to prevent bleeding and hematoma formation. (*C*) The periosteum is then closed with buried absorbable suture. The ulnar nerve can be seen here resting without tension over the previous location of the epicondyle.

- By placing the osteotome flush with the fibers of the collateral ligament, typically an amount of 5 to 7 mm of the epicondyle is removed while preserving the integrity of the medial collateral ligament. This amount is also enough to allow the ulnar nerve to easily glide past the epicondyle when the elbow is in a flexed position.
- Surgical outcomes following a minimal medial epicondylectomy have been found to achieve comparable outcomes to more aggressive epicondylectomies.[27]
- After skin closure, patients are placed in a soft dressing. The postoperative protocol is the same as for in situ release, with progression of activities as patients can tolerate.

Anterior Transposition

Three main techniques have been described for performing an anterior transposition: subcutaneous, intramuscular, and submuscular. All 3 techniques have the goal of removing both compressive and tensile effects on the nerve. As such, they all begin with a similar thorough decompression of the nerve.

- A sterile tourniquet is typically used, and an 8- to 17-cm incision is made between the medial epicondyle and the olecranon.
- The nerve is identified and dissected completely free of its surrounding sheath along the course of the incision, taking special care to decompress the arcade of Struthers proximally, the cubital tunnel, and superficial and deep layers of fascia at the FCU.
- The nerve is then circumferentially freed. A Penrose drain can be placed around the nerve to assist in gently mobilizing the nerve while this dissection is performed.
- In most cases, the extrinsic blood supply can be seen traveling with the nerve. Attempts should be made to perform the dissection while keeping these vessels with the nerve for a distance as distal as possible.
- Once the nerve is mobilized, the medial intermuscular septum should be identified and resected all the way down to the level

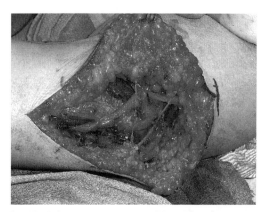

Fig. 10. Subcutaneous transposition: The ulnar nerve is seen coursing under a sling that has been constructed from the fascia of the flexor-pronator mass.

of the humerus for a distance of 4 to 5 cm. A large plexus of veins always travels through the septum just proximal to the epicondyle, and care should be taken to ligate or coagulate these vessels to prevent postoperative hematoma formation.

- At this point, the nerve should be mobilized anteriorly over the epicondyle. In many instances, the first motor branch to the FCU will tether the ulnar nerve and prevent a tensionless transposition. In such cases, the motor branch should be neurolysed proximally until the nerve can be easily transposed.
- Also after the nerve is transposed, efforts should be made to confirm that the nerve is lying without tension through a full range of elbow motion and without any points of constriction.

Subcutaneous

Several different techniques have been described for securing the nerve in an anterior position.

The easiest technique is to suture some of the subcutaneous tissue from the anterior skin flap down to the periosteum of the medial epicondyle. Others have advocated creating a fascial flap from the fascia covering the flexor-pronator mass (**Fig. 10**). After subcutaneous transposition, patients may be allowed immediate range of motion in a soft dressing. Activities can be progressed as tolerated.

Intramuscular

In an intramuscular transposition, once the nerve has been dissected free and the intermuscular septum removed, then the nerve is transposed anterior to the medial epicondyle and its course is noted. A skin marker can then be used to trace this course at a position about 2 cm anterior to the epicondyle. A scalpel is then used to cut the fascia along this line. The scalpel can then also be used to scrape the underlying muscle from the fascia both anteriorly and posteriorly. A trough is then made within the muscle and along the anticipated course of the nerve, taking special care to cut the fascial bands within the flexor-pronator mass to allow a wide path through which the nerve can travel. The nerve is then placed within the muscular bed, and the fascia is reapproximated with an absorbable suture, taking care to keep the proximal and distal apertures wide open so they do not constrict the nerve. After intramuscular transposition, patients are immobilized in a long-arm posterior splint for 2 weeks, and then transitioned to a removable splint. Activities are then slow progressed to full activity at 8 to 10 weeks.

Submuscular

Learmonth[28] initially described the submuscular transposition in 1942. Since then, variations on the technique have also been developed. In this technique, after the nerve is dissected throughout

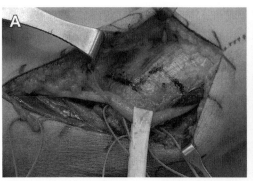

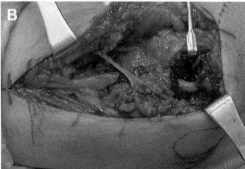

Fig. 11. Submuscular transposition. (*A*) The z lengthening is planned with a marking pen. (*B*) The ulnar nerve can be seen coursing under the z-lengthened flexor-pronator mass. Also note the distal crossing branch of the medial antebrachial cutaneous nerve. (*Courtesy of* Brian Fitzgerald, MD.)

Table 1
Summary of prospective comparative studies for surgical treatment of cubital tunnel syndrome

Authors	Year	N	Treatment Groups	Metrics	Results
Nabhan et al[30]	2005	66	In-situ v. SCUNT	physical exam, Yale sensory scale, Edx	No difference in any outcomes.
Bartels et al[31]	2005	152	In-situ v. SCUNT	SF-36, McGill Pain Questionnaire, Edx	Higher MABC related complication rate in SCUNT group. No difference in EMG or outcomes questionnaires.
Gervasio et al[32]	2005	70	In-situ v. SMUNT	Bishop Score, Edx	No difference in any outcomes.
Biggs & Curtis[33]	2006	44	In-situ v. SMUNT	McGowan class, LSUMC system	Higher rate of deep infection in SMUNT group (did not reach statistical significance). No difference in postop classification.

Abbreviations: Edx, electrodiagnostics; LSUMC, Louisiana State University Medical Center; MABC, medial antebrachial cutaneous nerve; SCUNT, subcutaneous ulnar nerve transposition; SF-36, Standard Form 36; SMUNT, submuscular ulnar nerve transposition.

its course, attention is directed to the flexor-pronator mass. The interval between the underlying ulna and the flexor-pronator mass is developed. The flexor pronator mass is divided, either straight across or in a step-cut fashion (**Fig. 11**A), and the mass is then lifted away from the bone and peeled distally to make an interval through which the nerve can travel. The nerve is then transposed as previously described, and the muscle is repaired with an absorbable suture either primarily or with the step-cut lengthened pattern (see **Fig. 11**B). Alternatively, Fitzgerald and colleagues[29] described lifting the flexor-pronator mass off the epicondyle subperiosteally to gain access to the submuscular interval. Once the nerve is transposed, the flexor-pronator mass is repaired back to the epicondyle with suture anchors. Postoperative care is the same as the intramuscular protocol.

AN EVIDENCE-BASED APPROACH TO SURGICAL DECISION MAKING

There are few high-level studies to help determine the best surgical treatment option for cubital tunnel syndrome. Universally, studies suggest that patients with more severe disease (McGowan III) at the time of surgery will not achieve the same results as those with milder disease.

To date, all prospective randomized studies suggest that there is no significant difference in patient outcomes when comparing in situ (simple) decompression with anterior transposition procedures, except with regard to complication rates. A summary of the only randomized prospective studies is presented in **Table 1**. When considering

this fact, it is reasonable to conclude (and it is also the author's opinion) that the preferred first-line treatment of patients with cubital tunnel syndrome should start with an in situ decompression. In the case of a subluxating ulnar nerve after in situ decompression, the surgeon should consider the addition of some additional procedure to allow for the decrease in tension of the nerve. This procedure could include either a medial epicondylectomy or some form of a formal anterior transposition.

SUMMARY

Cubital tunnel syndrome is a common condition. With knowledge of the ulnar nerve anatomy and clinical findings associated with the condition, the clinician can easily diagnose most cases. Electrodiagnostic testing can be helpful in more complex cases. A variety of surgical treatments are described to treat cubital tunnel, all of which yield reliable results in mild to moderate cases. Thus, the treatment of cubital tunnel syndrome is preferred in the earlier stages when possible.

REFERENCES

1. Panas J. Sur une cause peu connue de paralysie du nerf cubital. Arch Gen de Med 1878;2:5–15 [in French].
2. Heithoff S. Cubital tunnel syndrome does not require transposition of the ulnar nerve. J Hand Surg Am 1999;24:898–905.
3. Magee RB, Phalen GS. Tardy ulnar palsy. Am J Surg 1949;78:470–4.

4. Osborne GV. The surgical treatment of tardy ulnar neuritis [abstract]. J Bone Joint Surg Br 1957;39:782.

5. Feindel W, Stratford J. The role of the cubital tunnel in tardy ulnar palsy. Can J Surg 1958;1:287–300.

6. Palmer BA, Hughes TB. Cubital tunnel syndrome. J Hand Surg Am 2010;35:153–63.

7. Elhassan B, Steinmann SP. Entrapment neuropathy of the ulnar nerve. J Am Acad Orthop Surg 2007; 15:672–81.

8. Wiesler ER, Chloros GD, Cartwright MS, et al. Ultrasound in the diagnosis of ulnar neuropathy at the cubital tunnel. J Hand Surg Am 2006;31:1088–93.

9. Gervasio O, Zaccone C. Surgical approach to ulnar nerve compression at the elbow caused by the epitrochleoanconeus muscle and a prominent medial head of the triceps. Neurosurgery 2008; 62(3 Suppl 1):186–92.

10. Smith JW. Factors influencing nerve repair: II. Collateral circulation of peripheral nerves. Arch Surg 1966;93:433–6.

11. Ogata K, Manske PR, Lesker PA. The effect of surgical dissection on regional blood flow to the ulnar nerve in the cubital tunnel. Clin Orthop 1985; 193:195–8.

12. Prevel CD, Matloub HS, Ye Z, et al. The extrinsic blood supply of the ulnar nerve at the elbow: an anatomic study. J Hand Surg Am 1993;18:433–8.

13. Lowe JB, Maggi SP, MacKinnon SE. The position of the crossing branches of the medial antebrachial cutaneous nerve during cubital tunnel surgery in humans. Plast Reconstr Surg 2004;114:692–6.

14. Iba K, Wada T, Aoki M, et al. Intraoperative measurement of pressure adjacent to the ulnar nerve in patients with cubital tunnel syndrome. J Hand Surg Am 2006;31:553–8.

15. Gelberman RH, Yamaguchi K, Hollstein SB, et al. Changes in interstitial pressure and cross-sectional area of the cubital tunnel and of the ulnar nerve with flexion of the elbow: an experimental study in human cadavera. J Bone Joint Surg Am 1998;80: 492–501.

16. Hicks D, Toby EB. Ulnar nerve strains at the elbow: the effect of in situ decompression and medial epicondylectomy. J Hand Surg Am 2002;27:1026–31.

17. McGowan A. The results of transposition of the ulnar nerve for traumatic ulnar neuritis. J Bone Joint Surg Br 1950;32:293–301.

18. Dellon AL. Review of treatment results for ulnar nerve entrapment at the elbow. J Hand Surg 1989; 14(4):688–700.

19. Cheng CJ, Mackinnon-Patterson B, Beck JL, et al. Scratch collapse test for evaluation of carpal and cubital tunnel syndromes. J Hand Surg Am 2008;33: 1518–24.

20. Svernlov B, Larsson M, Rehn K, et al. Conservative treatment of the cubital tunnel syndrome. J Hand Surg Br 2009;34:201–7.

21. Bryon PM. Upper extremity nerve gliding: programs used at the Philadelphia Hand Center. In: Hunter JM, Mackin EJ, Callahand AD, editors. Rehabilitation of the hand: surgery and therapy. 4th edition. St Louis (MO): Mosby; 1995. p. 951–6.

22. Tsai RM, Bonczar M, Tsuruta T, et al. A new operative technique: cubital tunnel decompression with endoscope assistance. Hand Clin 1995;11:71–80.

23. Hoffman R, Siemionow M. The endoscopic management of cubital tunnel syndrome. J Hand Surg Br 2006;31:23–9.

24. Ahcan U, Zorman P. Endoscopic decompression of the ulnar nerve at the elbow. J Hand Surg Am 2007;32:1171–6.

25. Watts AC, Gain GL. Patient-rated outcomes of ulnar nerve decompression: a comparison of endoscopic and open in situ decompression. J Hand Surg Am 2009;34:1492–8.

26. King T. The treatment of traumatic ulnar neuritis; mobilization of the ulnar nerve at the elbow by removal of the medial epicondyle and adjacent bone. Aust N Z J Surg 1950;20:33–42.

27. Amako M, Nemoto K, Kawaguchi M, et al. Comparison between partial and minimal medial epicondylectomy combined with decompression for the treatment of cubital tunnel syndrome. J Hand Surg Am 2000;25:1043–50.

28. Learmonth JR. A technique for transplanting the ulnar nerve. Surg Gynecol Obstet 1942;75:792–3.

29. Fitzgerald BT, Dao KD, Shin AY. Functional outcomes in young, active duty, military personnel after submuscular ulnar nerve transposition. J Hand Surg Am 2004;29:619–24.

30. Nabhan A, Ahlhelm F, Kelm J, et al. Simple decompression or subcutaneous anterior transposition of the ulnar nerve for cubital tunnel syndrome. J Hand Surg Br 2005;30(5):521–4.

31. Bartels RH, Verhagen WI, vanderWilt GJ, et al. Prospective randomized controlled study comparing simple decompression versus anterior subcutaneous transposition for idiopathic neuropathy of the ulnar nerve at the elbow: part I. Neurosurgery 2005;56: 522–30.

32. Gervasio O, Gambardella G, Zaccone C, et al. Simple decompression versus anterior submuscular transposition of the ulnar nerve in severe cubital tunnel syndrome: a prospective randomized study. Neurosurgery 2005;56:108–17.

33. Biggs M, Curtis JA. Randomized, prospective study comparing ulnar neurolysis in situ with submuscular transposition. Neurosurgery 2006;58(2):296–304.

Evaluation and Treatment of Failed Ulnar Nerve Release at the Elbow

Kate Nellans, MD, MPH, Peter Tang, MD, MPH*

KEYWORDS

- Failed ulnar nerve release • Revision cubital tunnel syndrome release • Revision nerve surgery

KEY POINTS

- Failure after ulnar nerve decompression at the elbow can be defined as either no change in the patient's symptoms after surgery or an initial improvement with recurrence of symptoms.
- Failure may be attributable to diagnostic (incorrect diagnosis or coexistent diagnoses), technical (incomplete decompression, creation of a new area of compression or subluxation, or injury to the cutaneous or ulnar nerves), or biologic (perineural fibrosis or significant preoperative nerve damage) factors.
- Diagnosis must be verified with a basic history and physical examination ± further studies, such as a nerve study if one was not performed initially.
- Technical errors and the development of perineural fibrosis necessitate revision surgery, whereas nerve damage owing to chronic severe compression should be observed.
- No one procedure is superior in the revision setting as long as a complete decompression from the Arcade of Struthers to the flexor carpi ulnaris (FCU) and flexor/pronator aponeurosis is achieved with a compression-free, stable transposition of the surgeon's choice.

INTRODUCTION

Compression of the ulnar nerve around the elbow, also known as cubital tunnel syndrome, is the second most common compressive neuropathy in the upper extremity after carpal tunnel syndrome. Unlike carpal tunnel syndrome, however, there are multiple sites of compression as well as multiple surgical techniques with cubital tunnel syndrome. Surgical options include open in situ decompression, endoscopic decompression, anterior transposition (subcutaneous, intramuscular, submuscular), and medial epicondylectomy. The subsequent evaluation and treatment of a failed ulnar nerve decompression at the elbow remain similar to the evaluation and treatment for a new diagnosis of cubital tunnel syndrome, but the outcomes for this problem are more unpredictable.[1–4] Discussion of surgical treatment failure for cubital tunnel syndrome warrants defining the term "failure," and reviewing its causes and the optimal workup and treatment for this condition.

Defining Failures

Defining a surgical "failure" after a cubital tunnel release, with or without transposition, requires a standardized approach. The 2 main types of failures include (1) patient's symptoms are unchanged, and (2) patient's symptoms initially improved and then recurred (**Table 1**). Failure may be attributable to an error in diagnosis (incorrect

Department of Orthopaedic Surgery, New York Presbyterian Hospital, Columbia University, 622 West 168th Street, PH11, New York, NY 10032, USA
* Corresponding author.
E-mail address: pt2214@columbia.edu

Orthop Clin N Am 43 (2012) 487–494
http://dx.doi.org/10.1016/j.ocl.2012.07.018
0030-5898/12/$ – see front matter © 2012 Elsevier Inc. All rights reserved.

orthopedic.theclinics.com

Table 1
Types of failure in primary ulnar nerve decompression with etiologies, work-up, and treatment options

Patient Symptoms	Likely Etiologies	Workup	Treatment Options/ Recommendations
• No change in symptoms	• Incorrect diagnosis	• History and physical examination, nerve study (if one had not been done) or repeat study, cervical and/or wrist magnetic resonance imaging	• Treatment for secondary compression or alternative diagnosis
	• Incomplete decompression or new site of compression	• Consider repeat nerve study	• Revision decompression
	• Significant nerve damage before index procedure	• Repeat nerve study to document nerve improvement	• Patient counseling, observation
• Resolved, then recurred	• Perineural fibrosis	• Repeat nerve study	• Revision decompression

diagnosis or coexistent diagnoses), technique (incomplete decompression, creation of a new area of compression or subluxation, or injury to the cutaneous or ulnar nerves), or biologic (perineural fibrosis or significant preoperative nerve damage) factors (**Table 2**). All these causes of failure except for perineural fibrosis, will lead to unchanged symptomatology. Fibrosis may be the cause of symptom recurrence after a period of improvement after the initial operation.

Table 2
Reasons for failure of primary ulnar nerve release at the elbow

Diagnostic
• Incorrect diagnosis
• Coexisting sites of compression

Technical
• Inadequate decompression
• Creation of new sites of compression during transposition
• Persistent or new ulnar nerve subluxation/ instability
• Injury to ulnar nerve or medial antebrachial cutaneous nerves

Biologic
• Perineural fibrosis/cicatrix
• Chronic, severe distal sensory and motor changes
• Elbow stiffness

Incidence of Failed Decompression

In his review of more than 2000 patients undergoing ulnar nerve release, Dellon[5] found that nearly 90% of patients with moderate compression achieved excellent results, but 20% to 35% of patients with severe compression noted a recurrence or "worsening" symptoms. He did add that in recurrent cases, the most favorable results were achieved when an internal neurolysis was performed in addition to a submuscular transposition. Bartels[6] reported on more than 3100 surgeries in which patients with unchanged symptoms or worsening of neurologic deficits occurred in 10.9% of simple decompressions, 14.6% of subcutaneous transpositions, 10.0% of intramuscular transpositions, and 21.0% of submuscular transpositions. In a meta-analysis reviewing 903 cases, Mowlavi and colleagues[7] found that in moderate-staged patients, no one treatment was statistically superior, with a recurrence rate of 4% and total relief in 80% of patients with submuscular transposition; however, in the severe-staged, all modalities were noted to provide similarly poor results, with 25% recurrence with decompression alone or transposition.

Determining Cause of Initial Failed Release

Diagnostic factors

First, it must be considered that if there is little or no relief from the initial ulnar nerve release at the elbow that the pain and dysfunction are a result of another condition that causes ulnar nerve irritation or symptoms similar to ulnar nerve problems. If the surgery was based on clinical examination findings only, without a confirmatory electrodiagnostic study, the initial assumed diagnosis of an isolated cubital tunnel syndrome may be incorrect. Even if an electrodiagnostic study was performed, the reported diagnostic accuracy ranges from 20% to 100%.[8] Because conduction velocities are variable, there is no absolute sensory and motor conduction value that is diagnostic of ulnar neuropathy at the elbow.[8–11] Motor studies are clearly less useful in the evaluation of patients with absent or subtle examination findings.[12–16] A study by Britz and colleagues[8] found that in clinically mild cubital tunnel neuropathies, 73% had electromyography findings consistent with an ulnar neuropathy, but only 68% had findings at the elbow. Even in patients with "definite" clinical symptoms of cubital tunnel syndrome, abnormalities in sensory or mixed nerves identified only 86% as having an ulnar nerve problem.[17] In patients with more subtle clinical presentations, they found these abnormalities in only 68% of patients.

Alternative compressive neuropathic diagnoses
Distally, compression of the ulnar nerve at the Guyon canal by either a ganglion cyst or aneurysm can produce similar symptoms in the hand as compression at the elbow, although this is estimated to have a 20 times lower incidence than cubital tunnel syndrome.[18] Distinguishing between these either clinically or with nerve conduction studies may be difficult, as the motor nerve fibers to muscles in the forearm are often spared with compression at the elbow, whereas the motor and sensory fibers to the hand are more affected (which would also be affected by compression at the wrist).[15,19] Hypothenar hammer syndrome may also present with ulnar nerve symptoms of the hand, although the primary etiology is an injury to the ulnar artery, leading to cold ulnar-sided digits but the ulnar nerve may also be involved. The dysvascular digits may present as subjective numbness and tingling. A history of repetitive occupational trauma in which the heel of the hand is often used as a hammer, can help make this diagnosis.

Compression occurring at the C8 nerve root from arthritis, or much more rarely a Pancoast tumor, can affect fibers that distally become the ulnar nerve, which would mimic symptoms of cubital tunnel syndrome. History-taking that includes inquiring about neck and radicular symptoms, as well as physical examination maneuvers, such as the "Spurling" test will help make the diagnosis. An electrodiagnostic study will also aid in the diagnosis. Furthermore, patients may have

compression at the elbow and the cervical spine, which leads to the so-called, "double crush" phenomenon, in which release at the elbow would not allow for complete resolution of symptoms.[20] Compression of the neurovascular bundle at the superior thoracic outlet, which is known as thoracic outlet syndrome, can also mimic cubital tunnel syndrome. These patients present with pain in the arms and hand, which may also be similar to a burning sensation, as well as possible discoloration of the hand. Lastly, a failure to diagnosis ulnar nerve subluxation over the medial epicondyle as the cause of ulnar nerve symptoms will lead to continued problems if in situ decompression is performed and subluxation is not evaluated intraoperatively.

Alternative noncompressive neuropathic diagnoses
Raynaud disease or phenomenon may also cause tingling and pain in the hand, but the accompanying skin blanching and association with cold, helps to differentiate it from a compressive neuropathy. Usually Raynaud disease affects all the fingers but may be isolated to particular fingers, and if only the ring and small are involved, this can be confused with cubital tunnel syndrome. Other causes of ulnar nerve irritation at and distal to the elbow include medial epicondylitis and FCU tendonitis, respectively, which can continue after ulnar nerve release. Another diagnosis that should be kept in mind is brachial plexus neuritis (Parsonage-Turner syndrome), which usually resolves without intervention. This diagnosis is made when the history and examination reveal abnormalities of the median, radial, and ulnar nerves. Last, polyneuropathy attributable to diabetes or a neurologic condition may be mistaken for cubital tunnel syndrome. Again, an electrodiagnostic study will be helpful in making this diagnosis.

Technical factors
The technical factors that lead to failure include failure to fully decompress the nerve, creation of new sites of compression or ulnar nerve subluxation, and injury to branches of the medial antebrachial cutaneous nerve or the ulnar nerve itself.

Inadequate release Amadio[21] described 5 major anatomic sites of compression in cubital tunnel syndrome: the arcade of Struthers, the medial intermuscular septum, the medial epicondyle, the cubital tunnel, and the deep flexor pronator aponeurosis. In his case series of 41 patients, 3 had constriction at the arcade, 2 at the medial intermuscular septum, 13 at the region of the medial epicondyle, 17 at the cubital tunnel, and 4 at the distal flexor pronator aponeurosis, whereas 12 had no apparent constrictive focus. All these sites need to be considered when a revision is being considered. However, there have never been any large studies reporting the incidence of the location of compression in the primary setting, although the cubital tunnel and the 2 heads of the FCU are reported as the most common sites of compression. We consider the arcade of Struthers a potential site of compression if not resected with transposition, and it is unclear if it is ever a primary site of compression. Of note, Wehrli and Oberlin[22] believe that the arcade of Struthers should be called the internal brachial ligament, as Struthers originally described it in 1854. In this article, they felt the medial intermuscular septum is only a site of compression if it is not resected with transposition. As for the medial epicondyle, it is unclear to us how it is a primary site of compression. Other potential sites include a hypertrophied triceps, a dislocation (snapping) of the medial portion of the triceps,[23] an anomalous epitrochleo-anconeus muscle (also known as anconeus-epitrochlearis, subanconeus, or accessory anconeus),[24] and the ligament of Spinner, which is a distinct aponeurosis between the flexor digitorum superficialis of the ring finger and the humeral head of the FCU.[25]

Failures following incomplete decompression without transposition range from 6% to 20%.[5,26,27] Gabel and Amadio[2] found that during 30 revision cubital tunnel cases an average of 2.2 sites of compression were found: 24 had compression at the level of the medial epicondyle; 16 at the medial intermuscular septum; 13 at the cubital tunnel or the FCU arcade; and 7 at the arcade of Struthers and deep flexor pronator aponeurosis. Failure to recognize osteophytes at the medial epicondylar groove as a result of significant osteoarthritis may also result in incomplete decompression. Even if the overlying fascia is resected, the nerve may be compressed from within the floor of the cubital tunnel.[28]

Creation of new areas of compression Anterior transposition can move the nerve from the environment of the cubital tunnel and medial epicondyle, but can create other levels of mechanical impingement on the nerve. Kinking proximally at the arcade of Struthers or medial intramuscular septum, and distally at the fascial bands between the two heads of the FCU can lead to poor results after transposition. Subcutaneous transposition may uniquely leave the nerve exposed to external trauma, and the nerve has been frequently found directly overlaying the medial epicondyle at revision surgery.[29] A medial epicondylectomy is purported to potentially result in scarring and fibrosis from the exposed cancellous bone, which could lead to recurrent ulnar nerve symptoms.

As reported before, among 30 revisions, Gabel and Amadio[2] attributed the surgical failures to persistent compression at the medial intermuscular septum (16), cubital tunnel or FCU arcade (13), and the arcade of Struthers and deep flexor aponeurosis (7).[2] In 13 cases of previous transpositions, Rogers and colleagues[3] noted that the septum had been left intact in 12 cases. A severe kinking of the nerve over an unresected septum was observed in 6 of 10 cases by Filippi and colleagues,[1] whereas Caputo and Watson[30] reported an incompletely resected septum in 15 of 20 cases. Vogel and colleagues[4] found retained medial intermuscular septum (10), common flexor aponeurosis (9), and arcade of Struthers (5) as the cause of failure in their 18 patients who failed cubital tunnel surgery. Most recently, Mackinnon and Novak[29] found the most common site of compression in 100 revision cubital tunnel surgeries to be distally at the fascial septum between the FCU and the flexor/pronator muscle mass. In their study, it was twice as common at this site when compared to the site of the medial intermuscular septum.

Nerve subluxation The overall incidence of anterior instability in the setting of simple decompressions is cited to range from 2.4% to 17.0% of cases.[6] In 5 of 10 failures in the patients who had undergone decompression without transposition, it was found that dynamic subluxation was occurring with deep elbow flexion, which was assumed to be causing persistent irritation to the nerve.[31] Nerve instability was found in 8 patients in Vogel and colleagues'[4] case series of 18 patients. Additionally, in cases where an inadequate subcutaneous sling is constructed, the ulnar nerve has been noted to fall back into the epicondylar groove. We suggest closing the cubital tunnel after transposition to prevent this from occurring.[32]

Nerve injury Direct injury to the ulnar nerve, while rare, can be a catastrophic complication. More commonly, branches of the medial antebrachial cutaneous nerve are injured in the superficial dissection as they cross the incision within 6 cm proximal and distal to the medial epicondyle.[33] In Mackinnon and Novak's review of 100 failed ulnar nerve cases, they saw 73 medial antebrachial cutaneous neuromas, and felt this to be one of the major causes of failed decompression and transposition.[29] However, some would characterize this as a complication of the procedure and not a failure. Some patients could interpret their symptoms from the neuroma as similar to their preoperative ulnar nerve symptoms. Mackinnon and Novak[29] urged meticulous technique in the primary setting to prevent neuroma formation and electrocautery "capping" of excised neuroma nerve endings in the revision setting to prevent recurrence of painful neuromas. If the medial antebrachial cutaneous branch is injured, we would recommend primary repair using miscrosurgical technique.

Biologic factors

Perineural fibrosis Broudy and colleagues[34] found in 10 revision cases that scarring at the transposition site was frequent. Gabel and Amadio's[2] finding of an average of 2.2 sites of compression and its various locations, which were reviewed previously, were all described as fibrosis. Rogers and colleagues[3] reviewed 14 patients who had failed ulnar nerve release and found dense scarring of the nerve to the medial epicondylectomy site in 7, scarring in the cubital tunnel in the 1 patient who had in situ decompression, and 1 patient who had an intramuscular transposition had thick scarring within the flexor pronator mass. In a report of 22 patients who had revision ulnar nerve decompression surgery, Filippi and colleagues[1] attributed 14 of the failures to perineural fibrosis. They found this in cases of both simple decompressions as well as transpositions. In 20 patients, Caputo and Watson[30] found an average 1.9 sites of compression: FCU aponeurosis and deep flexor pronator mass (14), medial intermuscular septum (15), and the medial epicondyle (6). Vogel, and colleagues[4] reported on 18 patients in whom most (15) had subcutaneous transposition, and found the most common operative findings to be perineural scarring (16). Dagregorio and Saint-Cast[35] found in their 9 patients who failed a primary submuscular transposition, dense scarring at the fascialmuscular flap in all cases.

Preoperative nerve damage Another reason for a lack of improvement in symptoms is significant preoperative nerve damage from chronic compression. The patient may see the index procedure as a failure if there is no change in symptoms or the improvement is mild or negligible. These outcomes have to do with the status of the nerve and are largely out of the hands of the surgeon and patient. The surgeon must recognize the possibility of irreversible nerve damage, communicate this to the patient, and manage the patient's expectations. The patient needs to understand that in this setting complete recovery may not occur. Also, intrinsic muscle atrophy once present will most likely not recover. Most likely, the patient will experience some improvement in symptoms in terms of degree and areas involved, and function continues to improve beyond 2 years after surgery.[36] The goal

of surgery in chronic severe compression cases should be to prevent worsening of motor and sensory dysfunction and symptoms. Dellon[5] found that in cases of long-standing symptoms and severe deficits, the results of surgical treatment are not satisfactory regardless of the surgical technique, with fewer than 50% of severe cases experiencing significant sensory improvement and just 25% experiencing sensory improvement.

Elbow stiffness Results in the past following ulnar nerve release were complicated by elbow stiffness resulting from excessive postoperative immobilization. Although technically not a failure of the nerve release, postoperative elbow stiffness can affect the functional use of the arm. Mackinnon and Novak[29] argue that early elbow motion is essential to preventing recurrence by preventing scarring and additional sites of compression in the revision setting. Weirich and colleagues,[37] however, did not find differences in pain, muscle strength, or overall satisfaction in a randomized study of early motion versus delayed motion after primary subcutaneous transposition. Currently for simple decompressions, most surgeons immobilize only until the wound has healed, or not at all. If a submuscular transposition is performed and the flexor pronator mass is reflected and then repaired, however, some would immobilize to allow the repair to heal.

Work-up of Failed Ulnar Nerve Release

Understanding the patient's symptoms both before and after the initial surgery, including subtle difference in pain and parasthesias, will guide the appropriate workup. In cases of residual or recurrent pain, a thorough examination with the other differential diagnoses in mind must be performed. Starting proximally, provocative testing for cervical nerve root impingement (Spurling test and Lhermitte sign), and thoracic outlet maneuvers (Adson, Wright, and Roos stress test) should be evaluated. Along the course of the ulnar nerve, a Tinel that is moving distally from the site of the positive Tinel on initial presentation is a good prognostic sign of reinnervation. A Tinel at the Guyon canal can indicate compression occurring at this site, although it is much less common than at the elbow. Intact sensation of the dorsal ulnar hand (via the dorsal ulnar sensory branch) may help distinguish compression at the Guyon canal rather than at the elbow. Tenderness at the medial epicondyle or along the FCU may indicate medial epicondylitis or FCU tendonitis, respectively, rather than cubital tunnel syndrome.

The role of repeat electrodiagnostic studies remains controversial. Most agree that the clinical examination and the patient's symptoms should dictate treatment decisions. In difficult cases, however, a worsening nerve study may help confirm the need for reexploration, whereas an improving electrodiagnostic study can be reassuring. Cervical magnetic resonance imaging (MRI) may confirm a clinical diagnosis of cervical nerve root impingement, whereas a wrist MRI can confirm a cyst or mass in the Guyon canal. In terms of grading systems, to date none of the grading systems can completely capture the patient experience and in the revision setting where many factors come into play; these grading systems have little prognostic value.

Surgical Treatment

Revision nerve surgery is challenging, as tissue planes may be disrupted and the nerve may be encased in scar. The first step is to identify the nerve. To aid in accurate identification of the nerve, the prior incision should be extended, thereby allowing identification of the ulnar nerve in normal tissue planes. The dissection of the nerve should then be moved into the previous surgical field. If it remains difficult to dissect the nerve free from the surrounding scar tissue, we recommend including a cuff of scar tissue around the nerve to avoid damaging it.

When performing a revision release, we recommend a "maximally" invasive approach in which the nerve is fully exposed at all potential sites of compression from the arcade of Struthers to the 2 head of the FCU and the deep flexor pronator aponeurosis. This exposure and nerve dissection will most likely not allow the nerve to stay stable in its native location (assuming an in situ decompression was performed during the index operation), and it will therefore most likely need to be transposed if it has not been already. The best case scenario is if there is one focal area of perineural fibrosis or compression, which would explain the failure of the index operation, such as an unresected medial intermuscular septum after an anterior transposition. This is not always the case, however, as even during primary cubital tunnel surgery it is not always obvious where the compression is located. As Gabel and Amadio[2] (2.2 sites) and Caputo and Watson[30] (1.9 sites) showed in their case series, there is usually more than one site of compression found during the revision surgery.

As in primary cubital tunnel surgery, there is no one technique that has been definitively proven superior to the rest. Dellon stated, "that little more than personal bias is available for guidance in selecting treatment."[5] The same can be applied to revision cubital tunnel surgery. Different

investigators have reported results for various procedures for revision surgery, including simple neurolysis,[35] subcutaneous transposition,[30] intramuscular transposition,[38] and submuscular transposition.[2–4,34] Most revision case series have reported on and supported submuscular transposition for unclear reasons. We believe it may be partly because it is the most technically demanding operation, leaving no other procedure that is more complex or intricate to chose.[32] We agree with Caputo and Watson[30] when they reviewed the articles by Broudy and colleagues,[34] Gabel and Amadio,[2] and Rogers and colleagues,[3] and stated that, "the rationale behind choosing a submuscular versus subcutaneous transposition for revision procedure in the 3 previous reports is not well described."

We believe that success after revision surgery depends on finding and removing any external compression on the ulnar nerve and then placing the nerve in a stable bed with no subluxation. An environment that inhibits scar formation would be ideal but there is no proven method to inhibit this process. Some have suggested that vein wrapping may insulate the peripheral nerve from developing scar tissue.[39–44] If the index procedure was a minimally invasive approach, such as endoscopic or in situ release of just the cubital tunnel, then the nerve will be in its native location. Nerve subluxation should be assessed, as it may be the cause of the failure, after complete decompression of all the previously reviewed potential sites of decompression. As stated previously, after revision decompression, the nerve will most likely not be stable in its native location and will need to be transposed. Our preferred transposition is subcutaneous with the reasoning that no structure is placed over the nerve (ie, the fascia of the flexor-pronator mass or the whole mass itself as in the intramuscular and submuscular transposition, respectively) and the nerve has a large potential space: all the space anterior to the fascia of the anterior elbow deep to the subcutaneous adipose tissue.

If the index procedure was subcutaneous transposition and scarring at that site was the etiology of the compression, then external neurolysis with revision of the subcutaneous transposition (fascia to subcutaneous flap) is an option so that the nerve sits stably in the transposed state; however, conversion to intramuscular or submuscular can be performed also. Likewise, if a submuscular or intramuscular site is excessively scarred, moving it out of the scarred bed to a subcutaneous site may be reasonable. Although revision ulnar nerve surgery at the elbow will require some external neurolysis, we see no role for internal neurolysis, as it most likely will injure the nerve further. Others agree that internal neurolysis may cause ischemia and infarction of the ulnar nerve.[1,2]

SUMMARY

Diagnostic, technical, and biologic factors can contribute to failure after cubital tunnel surgery. The first 2 factors are under the control of the surgeon, and errors in these arenas should be minimized. Biologic factors such as perineural fibrosis, scar formation, and preoperative (to index procedure) permanent nerve dysfunction cannot be controlled, but recognizing pre-existing nerve damage and counseling the patient about realistic goals for the surgery is essential to manage expectations. The workup of failed ulnar nerve surgery includes verifying the diagnosis and obtaining a detailed history of the patient's symptoms before and after their index procedure. Often the decision for surgery will be based on the patient's continued or recurrent symptoms. Electrodiagnostic studies should be repeated and can aid in decision making for revision surgery. Submuscular transposition has the most support in the literature by way of case series but has not been shown to be superior to other techniques in a prospective, randomized trial. Rather than a particular technique, we advocate that a thorough and complete decompression be performed from the arcade of Struthers to the flexor pronator aponeurosis and the nerve be placed in a compression-free, stable anterior transposition of the surgeon's choice.

REFERENCES

1. Filippi R, Charalampaki P, Reisch R, et al. Recurrent cubital tunnel syndrome. Etiology and treatment. Minim Invasive Neurosurg 2001;44(4):197–201.
2. Gabel GT, Amadio P. Reoperation for failed decompression of the ulnar nerve in the region of the elbow. J Bone Joint Surg Am 1990;72(2):213–9.
3. Rogers MR, Bergreld TG, Aulicino PL. The failed ulnar nerve transposition: etiology and treatment. Clin Orthop Relat Res 1991;269:193.
4. Vogel RB, Nossaman BC, Rayan GM. Revision anterior submuscular transposition of the ulnar nerve for failed subcutaneous transposition. Br J Plast Surg 2004;57(4):311–6.
5. Dellon AL. Review of treatment results for ulnar nerve entrapment at the elbow. J Hand Surg 1989; 14A:688–700.
6. Bartels RH. History of the surgical treatment of ulnar nerve compression at the elbow. Neurosurgery 2001;49:391–400.
7. Mowlavi A, Andrews K, Lille S, et al. The management of cubital tunnel syndrome: a meta-analysis of clinical studies. Plast Reconstr Surg 2000; 106(2):327.
8. Britz GW, Haynor DR, Kuntz C, et al. Ulnar nerve entrapment at the elbow: correlation of magnetic resonance imaging, clinical, electrodiagnostic, and intraoperative findings. Neurosurgery 1996;38(3):458.
9. Hilburn JW. General principles and use of electrodiagnostic studies in carpal and cubital tunnel syndromes. With special attention to pitfalls and interpretation. Hand Clin 1996;12(2):205.
10. Lowe III JB, Mackinnon SE. Management of secondary cubital tunnel syndrome. Plast Reconstr Surg 2004;113(1):e1.
11. Steiner H, Von Haken M, Steiner-Milz H. Entrapment neuropathy at the cubital tunnel: simple decompression is the method of choice. Acta Neurochir 1996; 138(3):308–13.
12. Brown WF, Dellon AL, Campbell WW. Electrodiagnosis in the management of focal neuropathies: the "WOG" syndrome. Muscle Nerve 1994;17(11):1336–42.
13. Eisen A. Early diagnosis of ulnar nerve palsy. Neurology 1974;24(3):256–62.
14. Payan J. Electrophysiological localization of ulnar nerve lesions. J Neurol Neurosurg Psychiatr 1969; 32(3):208.
15. Stewart J. The variable clinical manifestations of ulnar neuropathies at the elbow. J Neurol Neurosurg Psychiatr 1987;50(3):252.
16. Tackmann W, Vogel P, Kaeser H, et al. Sensitivity and localizing significance of motor and sensory electroneurographic parameters in the diagnosis of ulnar nerve lesions at the elbow. J Neurol 1984; 231(4):204–11.
17. Raynor EM, Shefner JM, Preston DC, et al. Sensory and mixed nerve conduction studies in the evaluation of ulnar neuropathy at the elbow. Muscle Nerve 1994;17(7):785–92.
18. Kwak KW, Kim MS, Chang CH, et al. Ulnar nerve compression in Guyon's canal by ganglion cyst. J Korean Neurosurgical Society 2011;49(2):139.
19. Osborne G. Compression neuritis of the ulnar nerve at the elbow. Hand 1970;2(1):10–3.
20. Upton AR, Mccomas AJ. The double crush in nerve-entrapment syndromes. Lancet 1973;302(7825): 359–62.
21. Amadio PC. Anatomical basis for a technique of ulnar nerve transposition. Surg Radiol Anat 1986; 8(3):155–61.
22. Wehrli L, Oberlin C. The internal brachial ligament versus the arcade of Struthers: an anatomical study. Plast Reconstr Surg 2005;115(2):471.
23. Spinner RJ, O'Driscoll SW, Jupiter JB, et al. Unrecognized dislocation of the medial portion of the triceps: another cause of failed ulnar nerve transposition. J Neurosurg 2000;92(1):52–7.
24. Ho K, Marmor L. Entrapment of the ulnar nerve at the elbow. Am J Surg 1971;121(3):355–6.

25. Inserra S, Spinner M. An anatomic factor significant in transposition of the ulnar nerve. J Hand Surg 1986;11(1):80.

26. Manske PR, Johnston R, Pruitt DL, et al. Ulnar nerve decompression at the cubital tunnel. Clin Orthop Relat Res 1992;274:231.

27. Goldfarb CA, Sutter M, Martens E, et al. Incidence of re-operation and subjective outcome following in situ decompression of the ulnar nerve at the cubital tunnel. J Hand Surg Eur Vol 2009;34(3):379–83.

28. Kurosawa H, Nakashita K, Nakashita H, et al. Pathogenesis and treatment of cubital tunnel syndrome caused by osteoarthrosis of the elbow joint. J Shoulder Elbow Surg 1995;4(1):30–4.

29. Mackinnon SE, Novak CB. Operative findings in re-operation of patients with cubital tunnel syndrome. Hand 2007;2(3):137–43.

30. Caputo AE, Watson HK. Subcutaneous anterior transposition of the ulnar nerve for failed decompression of cubital tunnel syndrome. J Hand Surg 2000;25(3):544–51.

31. Antoniadis G, Richter HP. Pain after surgery for ulnar neuropathy at the elbow: a continuing challenge. Neurosurgery 1997;41(3):585.

32. Tang P, Nellans KW. Cubital tunnel syndrome—surgical treatment techniques. Operat Tech Orthop 2009;19(4):235–42.

33. Waugh RP, Zlotolow DA. In situ decompression of the ulnar nerve at the cubital tunnel. Hand Clin 2007;23(3):319–27.

34. Broudy A, Leffert R, Smith R. Technical problems with ulnar nerve transposition at the elbow: findings and results of reoperation. J Hand Surg 1978;3(1):85.

35. Dagregorio G, Saint-Cast Y. Simple neurolysis for failed anterior submuscular transposition of the ulnar nerve at the elbow. Int Orthop 2004;28(6):342–6.

36. Matsuzaki H, Yoshizu T, Maki Y, et al. Long-term clinical and neurologic recovery in the hand after surgery for severe cubital tunnel syndrome. J Hand Surg 2004;29(3):373–8.

37. Weirich SD, Gelberman RH, Best SA, et al. Rehabilitation after subcutaneous transposition of the ulnar nerve: immediate versus delayed mobilization. J Shoulder Elbow Surg 1998;7(3):244–9.

38. Kleinman WB. Cubital tunnel syndrome: anterior transposition as a logical approach to complete nerve decompression. J Hand Surg 1999;24(5):886–97.

39. Zyluk A, Deskur Z, Prowans P, et al. Post-traumatic painful ulnar nerve compression syndrome treated by wrapping the nerve with the vein: preliminary report. Chir Narzadow Ruchu Ortop Pol 1997;62(6):483 [in Polish].

40. Kokkalis ZT, Jain S, Sotereanos DG. Vein wrapping at cubital tunnel for ulnar nerve problems. J Shoulder Elbow Surg 2010;19(2):91–7.

41. Varitimidis SE, Vardakas DG, Goebel F, et al. Treatment of recurrent compressive neuropathy of peripheral nerves in the upper extremity with an autologous vein insulator. J Hand Surg 2001;26(2):296–302.

42. Varitimidis S, Riano F, Vardakas D, et al. Recurrent compressive neuropathy of the median nerve at the wrist: treatment with autogenous saphenous vein wrapping. J Hand Surg Br 2000;25(3):271–5.

43. Xu J, Sotereanos DG, Moller AR, et al. Nerve wrapping with vein grafts in a rat model: a safe technique for the treatment of recurrent chronic compressive neuropathy. J Reconstr Microsurg 1998;14:323–8.

44. Xu J, Varitimidis SE, Fisher KJ, et al. The effect of wrapping scarred nerves with autogenous vein graft to treat recurrent chronic nerve compression. J Hand Surg 2000;25(1):93–103.

Late Reconstruction of Ulnar Nerve Palsy

Hilton P. Gottschalk, MD[a], Randip R. Bindra, MD[b],*

KEYWORDS

- Ulnar nerve • Tendon transfer • Peripheral nerve injury • Palsy

KEY POINTS

- Ulnar nerve palsy results in significant loss of sensation and profound weakness, leading to a dysfunctional hand.
- A sound understanding of the anatomy of the different muscles and biomechanics of the potential transfers will ensure optimal results in treatment.
- This article reviews the clinical findings seen in both low and high ulnar nerve palsies, and reviews the surgical options for correcting certain motor and sensory deficits.

INTRODUCTION

Loss of ulnar nerve function leads to reduced dexterity and altered aesthetic appearance of the hand. Whereas the predominant cause of ulnar nerve palsy is traumatic in the Western world, systemic neurologic conditions such as leprosy still predominate in developing countries.[1–3] A sound understanding of the anatomy of the different muscles and biomechanics of the potential transfers will ensure optimal results in treatment.[2] The aims of this article are to: (1) briefly review the pertinent anatomy; (2) describe the functional deficits associated with both high and low ulnar nerve palsy; (3) discuss various reconstructive procedures for restoration of function, sensibility, and aesthetics to the hand.

ANATOMY

The ulnar nerve is the terminal branch of the medial cord. It largely consists of nerve fibers from C8 and T1 nerve roots, but may have contributions from C7 or higher.[4–7] In the upper arm, the ulnar nerve lies medial or posterior to the brachial artery and pierces the medial intermuscular septum at the mid portion of the arm at the arcade of Struthers.[1,8]

It lies anterior to the medial head of the triceps muscle and travels through the cubital tunnel at the level of the elbow to pass between the 2 heads of the flexor carpi ulnaris (FCU) (which it innervates).[1,7] The FCU is usually the first muscle innervated by the ulnar nerve. As it continues distally, it lays on the volar surface of the flexor digitorum profundus (FDP) and sends branches to the FDP of the small and ring fingers. The next main branch off the ulnar nerve is the dorsal sensory branch, which originates approximately 7 cm proximal to the radial styloid and provides sensation to the ulnar aspect of the hand.[1,7] At the level of the wrist, the nerve enters into Guyon canal with the ulnar artery. Here the nerve divides into deep and superficial branches. The superficial branch provides sensation to the small finger and ulnar half of the ring finger. The deep motor branch innervates the hypothenar muscles, the 2 medial lumbricals, all interossei, the adductor pollicis, and the deep head of the flexor pollicis brevis. The most distal motor branch innervates the first dorsal interosseous muscle.[1,6,7]

Anomalous ulnar nerve anatomy and innervation patterns have been described.[7,9,10] The location where the anomalous pattern occurs defines the type of innervation pattern (**Table 1**). A forearm

[a] Central Texas Pediatric Orthopedics, 1301 Barbara Jordan Boulevard, Suite 300, Austin, TX 78723, USA;
[b] Department of Orthopaedic Surgery and Rehabilitation, Loyola University Medical Center, 2160 South First Avenue, Maguire Center Suite 1700, Maywood, IL 60153, USA
* Corresponding author.
E-mail address: rbindra@lumc.edu

Orthop Clin N Am 43 (2012) 495–507
http://dx.doi.org/10.1016/j.ocl.2012.08.001
0030-5898/12/$ – see front matter © 2012 Elsevier Inc. All rights reserved.

Table 1
Anomalous nerve connections

Martin-Gruber Anastomosis (Forearm Ulnar-Median Communication)			
Type	**Occurrence (%)**	**Description**	**Innervated Muscles**
I	60	Motor branches from median nerve to ulnar nerve	Median muscles
II	35	Motor branches from median nerve to ulnar nerve	Ulnar muscles
III	3	Motor fibers from ulnar nerve travel with median nerve	Median muscles
IV	1	motor fibers from Ulnar nerve travel with median nerve	Ulnar muscles
Riche-Cannieu (palmar communications)		Anomalous connection between motor branch ulnar nerve and recurrent branch median nerve	

ulnar-median communication pattern is known as the Martin-Gruber connection.[9] When the anomalous communication occurs in the palm, it is termed the Riche-Cannieu connection. The motor branch of the ulnar nerve and the recurrent motor branch of the median nerve are connected with ulnar to median innervation.[7,10,11] By knowing both the normal and variant anatomy, one can explain the functional deficits seen in patients with ulnar nerve lesions.

ASSESSMENT

Before any treatment options are discussed, a thorough clinical evaluation of the patient is necessary. The characteristic clinical signs that reflect the motor loss, sensory loss, and level of injury in ulnar nerve palsy have been well described (**Table 2**).[1,12] Palsy of the ulnar nerve leads to multiple complex

deficiencies, and the clinical significance of these vary according to age, relative joint laxity, soft-tissue and skin elasticity, and individual functional demands.[12]

The incident that led to the ulnar nerve palsy should be fully evaluated. The level of injury and mechanism can affect the prognosis and treatment of these patients. Ulnar nerve palsies are classified into high and low levels, where the nerve is affected above or below the elbow, respectively. The deficit and presentation varies between the 2 types of lesions and is discussed later.

Additional assessment includes evaluating the skin and soft tissues for any trophic ulcers occurring from sensory loss. A checklist of functioning and nonfunctioning muscles is created to better define the injury and availability of tendon transfers, especially for patients in whom the median nerve may be also be involved. In keeping with

Table 2
Clinical signs seen in ulnar nerve palsy

Clinical Sign	Description
Duchenne sign	Clawing deformity of fingers
Jeanne sign	Hyperextension of the thumb MCP joint during pinch
Froment sign	Thumb IP joint hyperflexion with pinch
Masse sign	Flattened metacarpal arch and hypothenar atrophy
Andre-Thomas sign	Worsening of claw deformity when patient attempts to extend fingers by flexing the wrist (tenodesis effect)
Pollock sign	High ulnar nerve palsy, inability to flex DIP joint of ring and small fingers secondary to loss of flexor digitorum profundus to the respective digits
Pitres-Testut sign	Inability to abduct the middle finger radially and ulnarly
Wartenberg sign	Abducted small finger (inability to adduct extended small finger)
Earle-Valstou sign	Inability to cross the index and middle fingers

Abbreviations: DIP, distal interphalangeal; IP, interphalangeal; MCP, metacarpophalangeal.

general principles of tendon transfers, all joints should be supple and deformities passively correctable.

The complex interaction between the intrinsic and extrinsic muscles becomes uncoupled as a result of intrinsic muscle paralysis, leading to clawing of the fingers. The unopposed pull of the long extensors leads to the metacarpophalangeal (MCP) joint assuming a position of hyperextension with the interphalangeal joints assuming a flexed position resulting from normal tension in the long flexor muscles, the so-called claw hand. As median innervated intrinsics are intact, the clawing is restricted to the ulnar 2 digits. Ironically, with a high ulnar palsy (and more muscle loss) the lack of flexor tone in the ulnar FDP results in a less severe claw, referred to as the "ulnar paradox." Over time, the deformity worsens as the MCP volar plate stretches along with attenuation of the central slip of the extensor apparatus, and the proximal interphalangeal (PIP) capsuloligamentous complex contracts, leading to fixed claw deformity. To assess the integrity of the extensor apparatus at the PIP joint, the Bouvier maneuver (**Fig. 1**) is performed. This maneuver involves passively stabilizing the MCP joint in flexion and asking the patient to actively extend the PIP joint. A positive maneuver is the demonstration of active extension of the PIP, which indicates an intact and functioning central slip. Any stiffness at the PIP joint requires a period of stretching and serial splinting through therapy and fitting of an orthotic device (**Fig. 2**).

DEFICITS AND TREATMENT

There are various functional deficits and various treatment options available to address them.

Aesthetic

With time, muscle atrophy leads not only to functional deficits but also changes the appearance of the hand. Muscle wasting is noticeable in the interosseous spaces and is most apparent in the first web space, and can be disconcerting to some patients. Although not routinely required, injection of dermal fillers such as fat autograft obtained by liposuction may be considered to fill subdermal defects in the interosseous spaces on the dorsum of the hand.[13–15]

Sensory

Sensation is lost in ulnar nerve palsy over the palmar side of the small finger and the ulnar half of the ring finger. In high ulnar nerve palsy, additional sensory loss over the dorsoulnar aspect of

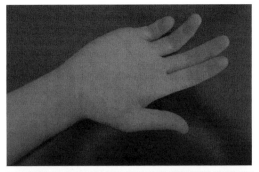
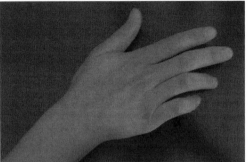
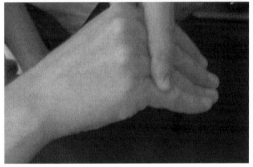

Fig. 1. Demonstration of the Bouvier maneuver. This maneuver involves passively stabilizing the MCP joint in flexion and asking the patient to actively extend the PIP joint. A positive maneuver is the demonstration of active extension of the PIP, which indicates intact and functioning central slip.

the hand is also observed. Loss of protective sensation along the ulnar border of the hand can be problematic in some patients who may be prone to injuring or burning their hands as a result of their occupation or hobbies.[7] In addition, the absence of sensation on the tip of the small finger can lead to skin breakdown and infections from minor repetitive trauma that is neglected.[16] Most patients can cope with the diminished sensibility by compensating with visual feedback, but if some patients develop recurrent injuries owing to the sensory loss, surgical intervention with sensory nerve transfer can be considered. Bertelli[16] has described using cutaneous branches of the median nerve to the palm as well as the palmar

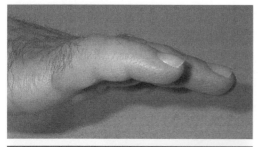

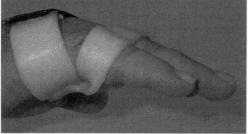

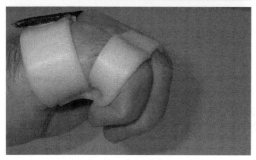

Fig. 2. Orthotic device donned to allow for extension of the PIP joint of the small finger.

cutaneous branch of the median nerve. The cutaneous nerves are transferred to the ulnar proper digital nerve of the small finger. Another option is to transfer the radial digital nerve of the middle finger (branch of the median nerve) (**Fig. 3**) or radial digital nerve of the ring finger to the ulnar proper digital nerve of the small finger.[17]

Motor

Muscles and subsequent movements that are affected in ulnar nerve palsy are listed in **Box 1**.

Low palsy

1. All interossei and ulnar 2 lumbricals resulting in loss of dexterity, weakness of grip, and clawing of ulnar 2 digits.
2. Adductor pollicis leading to weakness in key pinch.

High palsy
In lesions of the ulnar nerve above the elbow, in addition to aforementioned muscles, the following muscles and movements are also involved:

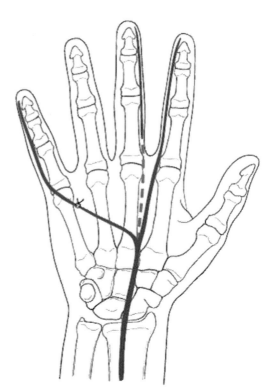

Fig. 3. Restoring sensation to the contact bearing edge of the small finger by transferring the radial digital nerve of the middle finger.

1. FCU, with weaker flexion and ulnar deviation of the wrist
2. FDP to the ring and small fingers, with loss of ring-finger and small distal interphalangeal (DIP) joint flexion.

Partial Loss of Wrist Flexion

Contraction of the FCU along with its counterpart on the extensor aspect of the wrist helps to stabilize the hand in power grip. Patients with loss of FCU activity do not observe any notable deficit with wrist motion, and reconstruction is not required. In special circumstances where ulnar deviation of the wrist is considered essential, the flexor carpi radialis innervated by the median nerve can be transferred to the FCU tendon.

Loss of Ring-Finger and Small DIP Joint Flexion (Weakness of Grasp)

In high ulnar nerve palsy, grasp is weakened approximately 60% to 80% secondary to loss of contraction in the ulnar half of the flexor profundus in addition to the loss of intrinsic function.[12] Lack of ability to close the ulnar side of the palm in forceful grip leads to difficulty with firmly holding on to objects. Restoration of flexion at the DIP

Box 1
Deficits in low and high ulnar nerve palsy

Low Ulnar Nerve Palsy (Below-Elbow Injury)

Loss of:

   Sensation small finger and ulnar half of ring finger

   Palmaris brevis

   Hypothenar musculature

      Abductor digiti minimi

      Flexor digiti minimi brevis

      Opponens digiti mini

   Ulnar 2 lumbricals

   Dorsal and volar interossei

   Adductor pollicis

   Deep head of flexor pollicis brevis

Clawing more pronounced because flexor digitorum profundus still innervated further proximally

High Ulnar Nerve Palsy (Above-Elbow Injury)

Includes low ulnar nerve palsy deficits plus:

   Loss of ring- and small-finger flexor digitorum profundus

   Loss of flexor carpi ulnaris

   Loss of sensation dorsoulnar portion of hand

Clawing less pronounced because ring and small finger flexor digitorum profundus not functioning, hence no DIP joint flexion

Abbreviation: DIP, distal interphalangeal.

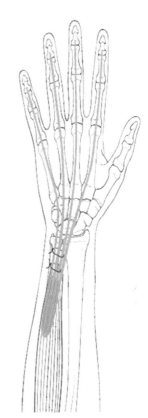

Fig. 4. Adjacent suturing of ring- and small-finger flexor digitorum profundus to middle-finger flexor digitorum profundus to restore flexion of the distal interphalangeal joint in ulnar nerve palsy.

joints of the ring and small fingers can be most easily achieved by adjacent suturing of the FDP tendons to the median innervated middle FDP tendon at the level of the distal forearm (**Fig. 4**).[7,12] The index-finger FDP tendon is not included, to preserve its independent function. As mentioned earlier, once flexor tone is restored to the ulnar 2 digits, the patient may note increased apparent clawing of the digits and should be forewarned about this paradox.

Clawing

Clawing is a result of a combination of lack of MCP flexion and PIP extension, both essentially served by the intrinsics in the hand. In simple clawing with positive Bouvier maneuver, maintaining the MCP joint in flexion with a passive tenodesis or active tendon transfer will suffice to correct the clawing.[1,7,12] The various options for claw correction are summarized in **Table 3** and include

bony procedures, soft-tissue tightening, and tendon transfers.

Static procedures

Several static procedures have been described with the intent of preventing MCP hyperextension:

1. Bony blocks on the dorsum of the metacarpal head[18]
2. MCP joint capsulodesis with volar plate advancement[19]
3. Bunnell[20] "flexor pulley advancement" to create bowstringing of flexor tendon
4. Tendon graft sutured to the deep transverse intermetacarpal ligament[21]

   Although some of these techniques are attractive because of their simplicity and ease of retraining, they do not add any power to grip and have the potential to lose correction as they stretch over time.

Dynamic

The authors prefer to use dynamic tendon transfers (**Table 4**), even in simple clawing. There are a few basic tenets for active restoration of intrinsic

Table 3
Static procedures for correction of claw deformity

Technique	Description	Comments
Bony Block		
Dorsal bony block (Mikhail)	Dorsally placed bone to block MCP hyperextension	Can be used in long-standing clawing with absent intrinsic function and weak extrinsic muscles
Static techniques		
Flexor pulley advancement (Bunnell)	Splitting of the proximal pulley system up to the mid portion of the proximal phalanx to allow bowstringing	Not effective if extensor apparatus damaged
Fasciodermadesis (Zancolli)	Excising 2 cm of palmar skin at MCP joint level combined with shortening of pretendinous band of palmar aponeurosis	Unable to prevent recurrence
Volar capsulodesis (Zancolli)	Release of A1 pulley with MCP joint volar plate advancement	Spares available motors to restore other important functions. Grip strength not augmented, recurrence has been reported
Static Tenodesis Techniques		
ECRL and ECU grafts (Riordan)	One half of ECRL and ECU tendons are used as grafts to prevent hyperextension of MCP joint while the remaining portion continues to actively extend the wrist	ECU can be used alone if only ring and small fingers involved
Volar side free tendon grafts (Parkes)	Free tendon grafts from (PL, plantaris, or toe extensor) connects the flexor retinaculum to the radial side of the dorsal extensor apparatus over PIP joint	Corrects clawing and allows grafts to function independent of the wrist. Does not restore metacarpal flexion

Abbreviations: ECRL, extensor carpi radialis longus; ECU, extensor carpi ulnaris; MCP, metacarpophalangeal; PIP, proximal interphalangeal; PL, palmaris longis.

function in the hand that do not change, regardless of the motor muscle used:

1. Tendon transfer must be passed volar to the transverse metacarpal ligament (acting as a pulley) to create the flexion moment at the MCP joint.
2. The tendon transfer is inserted onto the proximal phalanx directly into bone or flexor sheath, or is woven into the extensor apparatus at the level of the lateral bands.
3. The more distal the insertion the greater is the moment arm leading to better MCP flexion.
4. Insertion into the extensor apparatus will result in both MCP flexion and PIP extension, more closely mimicking the intrinsic function. However, overtensioning the transfer in patients with joint laxity can result in a swan-neck deformity.

Three main types of dynamic procedures have been described: (1) dynamic tenodesis,[22,23] whereby a tendon is looped through the extensor retinaculum, along the lumbricals, and inserted into the lateral bands; (2) dynamic procedures using digital flexors; and (3) dynamic procedures powered by wrist motors (extensor carpi radialis brevis, extensor carpi radialis longus, or flexor carpi radialis).

Flexor digitorum superficialis transfer for clawing

Using the sublimus tendon of the ring or middle finger is an attractive option to correct clawing because the donor is relatively easy to harvest, the length of tendon is adequate without the need for extension with a free graft, and because incisions are concealed on the palmar surface the clawing is corrected without additional aesthetic compromise. The main disadvantage of using superficialis transfers is that although they reliably correct clawing, they do not improve grip

Table 4
Dynamic procedures for correction of claw deformity

Technique	Description	Comments
Dynamic Tenodesis Wrist tenodesis (Fowler and Tsuge)	Free tendon graft attached to central extensor retinaculum and passed from dorsal to palmar, deep to DTML and inserted into lateral bands	Tenodesis loosens with time
Extrinsic Finger Flexors Flexor digitorum superficialis (modified Stiles-Bunnell)	Middle-finger FDS split into 4 slips, routed through lumbrical canal of each finger volar to the DTML, sutured to the lateral band of the extensor apparatus	Modified several times. PIP and DIP extension lag can occur in donor finger
Modifications of insertion sites Lateral band (Stiles, Bunnell) Phalangeal insertion (Burkhalter) Pulley insertion (Riordan, Zancolli) Interosseous insertion (Zancolli, Palande)		
Finger-Level Extensors Extensor indicis proprius and extensor digiti minimi (Fowler)	EIP and EDM tendons are transferred to lateral bands of dorsal apparatus	May produce excessive tension in extensor apparatus (intrinsic-plus deformity) and reverse metacarpal arch. Does not add grip strength
Wrist-Level Motor Transfers Dorsal route ECRB (Brand)	ECRB lengthened by free tendon graft (split into 4 tails); passed through intermetacarpal spaces, deep to DTML and attached to radial lateral bands MF, RF, SF, and ulnar lateral band IF	Does not improve metacarpal arch or grip strength. ECRL also used
Flexor carpi radialis (Riordan)	Flexor carpi radialis is augmented with free tendon graft brought around the forearm and then routed in similar fashion as described above by Brand	Removes FCR, strong wrist flexor
Flexor route ECRL (Brand)	Free tendon graft is passed through the carpal tunnel (split into 4 tails), and ECRL is used as the motor and brought around the forearm to the volar side	Uses free tendons for length (adhesions), Requires extensive therapy postoperatively, possible crowding of carpal tunnel can occur

Abbreviations: DTML, deep transverse metacarpal ligament; ECRB, extensor carpi radialis brevis; ECRL, extensor carpi radialis longus; EDM, extensor digitorum minimi; EIP, extensor indicis proprius; FCR, flexor carpi radialis; IF, index finger; MF, middle finger; RF, ring finger; SF, small finger.

strength, and may even result in decreased grip strength.[7,24] Another potential drawback in patients with lax joints is the potential for swan-neck deformity in the ring finger owing to the muscle imbalance created when the prime flexor is removed and used to augment the extensor apparatus.[25] Several variations of the flexor digitorum superficialis (FDS) transfer to correct clawing have been described.[24,26–31] The consistent part of the procedure is that the transferred tendon must be maintained volar to the deep intermetacarpal ligament. The decision regarding which finger FDS tendon to use depends on the level of the injury. The FDS to the ring fingers should not be used in high ulnar nerve palsy because it is the only functioning digital flexor. In patients with dynamic clawing of all fingers, consideration may be given to transfer to all 4 digits, although this is not necessary in most cases of isolated ulnar nerve palsy.

In the modified Stiles-Bunnell procedure,[7,20,29] the middle-finger FDS tendon is divided distally at its insertion and retrieved in the palm. The transfer has evolved from using all FDS tendons and transferring them to both sides of the affected digits to now using 1 FDS tendon to motor 2 adjacent digits (**Fig. 5**). The FDS tendon is divided through a transverse incision at the PIP joint crease and retrieved through a transverse incision in the palm at the distal palmar crease at the level of the A1 pulley. The preexisting split in the tendon is developed further proximally, and each slip is then passed on the radial side of the ring and small fingers along the path of the lumbrical, volar to the deep transverse metacarpal ligament where it is delivered through a supplementary incision along the midlateral line over the base of the proximal phalanx. The transferred tendon may be inserted in various ways and depends on the condition of the extensor mechanism as follows. In most cases, the tendon is woven into the lateral band of the extensor apparatus to simulate lumbrical action. In patients with a positive Bouvier maneuver and PIP joint laxity, to avoid secondary swan-neck deformity the transfer can be anchored directly into the lateral aspect of the proximal phalanx by periosteal suture, drill hole, or bone anchor. In cases where the extensor mechanism

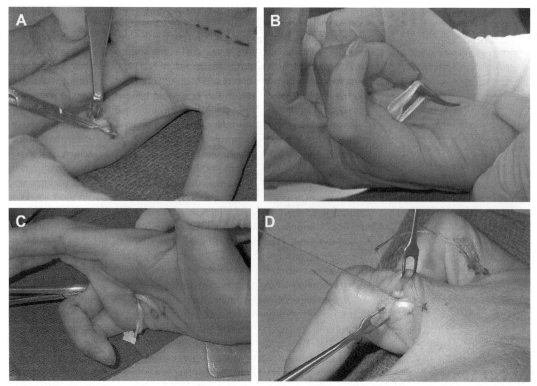

Fig. 5. Flexor digitorum superficialis (FDS) transfer to correct clawing. (*A, B*) The FDS tendon is divided through a transverse incision at the PIP joint crease and (*C*) retrieved through a transverse incision in the palm at the distal palmar crease at the level of the A1 pulley. (*D*) Each slip is passed on the radial side of the ring and small fingers along the path of the lumbrical, volar to the deep transverse metacarpal ligament, and then woven into the lateral band of the extensor apparatus to simulate lumbrical action.

is stretched and lax, the tendon is routed along the lateral band but secured into the central tendon so as to take up the slack in the extensor apparatus and provide better PIP extension. With the wrist in about 30° of flexion, the transferred tendon is tensioned so as to provide about 60° of MCP flexion.

The Zancolli[19] "lasso" procedure uses the FDS tendon to create a dynamic flexion tether for the MCP joint. The procedure is simple, and dissection is kept to the palm but requires the presence of a positive Bouvier maneuver because it does not add any extension power to the extensor apparatus.[19] In patients with PIP hyperextension, the distal stump of the FDS can be tenodesed to the proximal phalanx to prevent secondary swan-neck deformity. A single transverse incision is made across the MCP flexion crease in the palm and the A1 and proximal portion of the A2 pulleys are exposed, protecting the neurovascular bundles. The proximal and distal limits of the A1 pulley are identified at the base of each digit. Tension is applied to each A1 pulley to test if traction on the pulley will flex the MCP joint. Usually

the proximal portion of the A2 pulley has to be included for looping the FDS transfer. The sheath is opened transversely at approximately the proximal third of the A2 pulley and the FDS tendon is delivered into the wound. Both slips of FDS are divided as far distally as possible and the proximal portion of the slips is delivered into the wound. The 2 slips of FDS are then looped proximally volar to the flexor sheath and sutured back to the FDS tendon itself to create a 30° flexion at the MCP joint (**Fig. 6**). The ring-finger tendon can be split proximally using the ulnar slip for the small finger. Like the FDS transfer procedure, this transfer does not add strength to the hand.

Wrist motor tendon transfer for clawing

Several wrist motors have been used to correct digital claw deformity.[31–33] The advantage of using wrist tendon transfers over the FDS transfers is augmentation of grip strength and preservation of FDS function, minimizing the risk of swan-neck deformity. The procedure is more complex, however, as the tendon has to be lengthened with a free graft from the palmaris or plantaris

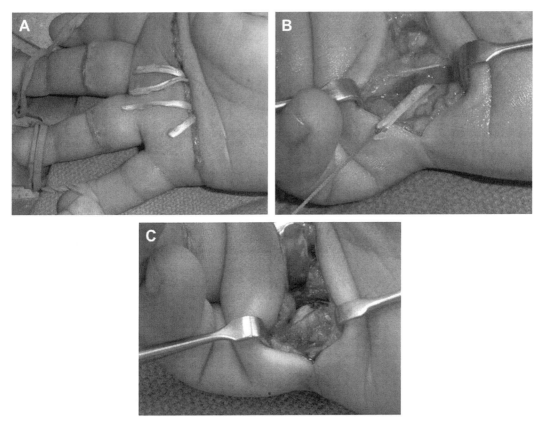

Fig. 6. Zancolli lasso technique for claw deformity correction. (*A*) Transverse incisions at the PIP joint and one across the palm to harvest FDS tendons. (*B*) FDS slip and A1 pulley is shown. (*C*) FDS tendon slips then looped proximally, volar to the flexor sheath and sutured back to the FDS tendon itself to create a 30° flexion at the MCP joint.

and has to be rerouted across the wrist and MCP joints. Flexor carpi radialis routed through the carpal tunnel[27] and the extensor carpi radialis brevis (ECRB) tendon routed subcutaneously across the dorsum of the wrist[31] have been described. The ECRB transfer is more commonly used, especially in combined median and ulnar palsy, as the wrist flexors are also affected. Through a dorsal incision, the ECRB tendon is released from its insertion and lengthened with a free tendon graft. The tendon graft is woven into the donor tendon at its midpoint, creating two "tails," one for each digit. An incision is made over the midlateral aspect on the radial side of each of the ring and small fingers, and the lateral band of the extensor is identified. With the hand supported in a closed-fist position, a straight hemostat is passed along the lumbrical canal in a retrograde direction, volar to the intermetacarpal ligament, to emerge at the longitudinal incision on the dorsum of the hand. Each slip of the lengthened donor tendon is then grasped and pulled through and is delivered in the digital incision, where it is woven into the lateral band. If the transfer is required for all 4 fingers, 2 free tendon grafts are necessary to create 4 tendon slips, 1 for each finger. In addition, the slip to the index finger is routed along its ulnar side to prevent index abduction, and provides better digital approximation when making a fist.

An alternative is to route the extensor carpi radialis longus (ECRL) tendon around the radial border of the forearm and to the fingers through the carpal tunnel. This maneuver has the advantage of providing a better vector for stronger finger flexion, but it can crowd the carpal tunnel (possibly causing carpal tunnel syndrome) and may create a wrist flexion deformity.[34,35] The authors' preference is a dorsal approach using the ECRB tendon extended with a doubled palmaris longus to create 2 slips going to the small and ring fingers.

Loss of Key Pinch

Key pinch requires forceful approximation of the tip of the thumb to the radial border of the index finger. It is the result of combined first dorsal interosseous and adductor pollicis function. Other extrinsic (extensor pollicis longus, flexor pollicis longus) and intrinsic (flexor pollicis brevis) muscles that contribute to key pinch remain intact with an ulnar palsy, and the focus in late reconstruction is to restore the function of the adductor pollicis, because the index finger can be stabilized against the adjacent fingers, compensating for the loss of the first dorsal interosseous.

Several different types of transfers have been described with different tendons acting as motors:

wrist extensors, brachioradialis, digital extensors, and digital flexors.[1,7,12,33,36–40] Regardless of the motor used, only 25% to 50% of normal pinch strength is restored.[1,12] Fortunately, not all patients with ulnar nerve palsy will have a noticeable loss of key pinch either from compensatory action of the flexor pollicis longus (Froment sign) or anomalous innervation of the adductor pollicis by the median nerve. It is therefore important to evaluate the need for transfer to restore thumb adduction in each patient on an individual basis.

Restoration of adductor pollicis function

The more commonly used tendon transfers for restoration of adductor pollicis function include FDS,[38–40] extensor digitorum communis,[36] ECRB,[37] and brachioradialis.[36] Finger flexors and extensors have been used to recreate the adductor pollicis function, but tend to have some disadvantages:

1. The direction of pull does not replicate that of the adductor pollicis
2. Harvesting of the FDS can further weaken grip strength
3. Finger extensor transfers are generally weak and have suboptimal vectors of pull[7]

Wrist extensors and the brachioradialis are strong donor muscle tendon units with no noticeable functional loss when harvested. The common factors with use of wrist motors include:

1. The need for a tendon graft to obtain appropriate length
2. Routing of the tendon between the second and third metacarpals into the palm. By using the second metacarpal as a pulley, the transfer is oriented in line with the original direction of pull of the adductor pollicis[37]

Extensor carpi radialis brevis transfer for thumb adduction

Smith[37] described using the ECRB tendon with a graft to restore thumb adduction. The distal end of the ECRB tendon is harvested just proximal to its insertion through a dorsal transverse incision at the wrist (**Fig. 7**). The tendon is then retrieved and delivered through a separate dorsal, transverse incision proximal to the extensor retinaculum. Two additional incisions are created on the hand, one over the ulnar side of the thumb MCP joint and one on the dorsal surface over the second web space. A tendon graft (usually palmaris longus) is sutured to the adductor pollicis insertion, and the proximal portion of the tendon graft is tunneled from palmar to dorsal deep to the adductor pollicis and through the window between

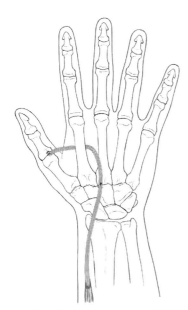

Fig. 7. Transfer of extensor carpi radialis brevis to adductor pollicis insertion to restore key pinch in ulnar nerve palsy.

the second and third metacarpals. The tendon graft is then woven into the ECRB tendon superficial to the extensor retinaculum. Tension is set so that the thumb lies just palmar to the index finger when the wrist is in neutral.

This technique has been modified by Omer[34] in 2 ways: (1) the tendon graft is passed through the intermetacarpal space between the third and fourth metacarpals; and (2) the graft is routed over the dorsum of the thumb and sutured to the fascia over the abductor tubercle of the thumb metacarpal, to provide better pronation for pinch.[1]

Brachioradialis transfer for thumb adduction

The brachioradialis can also be used as a motor.[36] An incision is made from the first dorsal compartment to the mid forearm to allow for mobilization of the tendon and its muscle belly, as the muscle has to be released from fascial attachments up to the proximal third of the radius to increase its excursion.[41] The brachioradialis tendon requires lengthening with a graft and is passed in the same manner as with the ECRB tendon.

Restoration of index abduction (first dorsal interosseous)

Most patients can stabilize the index finger by bracing it against adjacent fingers in pinch; however, a more versatile and stronger grasp can be achieved by restoring index-finger abduction.[37] The preferred method to restore the function of the first dorsal interosseous muscle is to transfer the accessory slip of the abductor pollicis

longus along with a tendon graft.[42] A dorsal radial incision is made over the first dorsal interosseous, and a dorsal subcutaneous path is made. The graft is woven into the insertion of the first dorsal interosseous at the base of the proximal phalanx of the index finger. The extensor indicis proprius tendon (which remains at the dorsal ulnar aspect of the joint) balances the index finger against this new abduction force and is able to reposition the deviated finger.[37]

Small-Finger Abduction (Wartenberg Sign)

Small-finger abduction results from paralysis of the third volar interosseous, which then leads to unopposed pull of the extensor digiti minimi (EDM). It has been postulated that this deformity may also be the result of reinnervation of the abductor digiti minimi but not the third volar interosseous.[43] The authors' preferred method of correction of small-finger abduction involves transferring the EDM (**Fig. 8**) to the radial aspect of the small finger.[44,45]

If there is no clawing evident, then the correction can be achieved by transferring the entire EDM tendon to the radial side of the extensor digitorum communis or to the radial lateral collateral ligament of the MCP joint.[44,46] If clawing is present, the tendon transfer can be used to perform both MCP flexion and digital adduction. The ulnar half of the EDM tendon is harvested at the distal edge of the extensor retinaculum. A separate palmar incision is made obliquely from the distal palmar crease overlying the MCP joint of the small

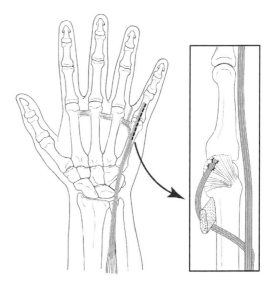

Fig. 8. Small-finger abduction deformity can be corrected with extensor digiti minimi (EDM) transfer to the radial aspect of the small finger.

Table 5
Ulnar nerve palsy: authors' preferred techniques

Deficit	Preferred Technique
Low Ulnar Palsy	
Sensory	If warranted, transfer of radial digital nerve middle finger to ulnar proper digital nerve small finger
Clawing	Extensor carpi radialis brevis and graft to small and ring fingers
Key pinch	Brachioradialis and graft passed through second to third metacarpal interspace to adductor pollicis tendon
Small-finger abduction	Transfer distal ulnar portion of EDM through fourth to fifth metacarpal interspace, then volar to DTML and inserted on radial aspect of proximal phalanx
High Ulnar Palsy	
As above for clawing, key pinch, and small-finger abduction	
Weak first dorsal interosseous	Transfer accessory slip APL with graft into first dorsal interosseous at base of proximal phalanx of index finger
Finger flexion	Side-to-side FDP middle to FDP ring and small fingers

Abbreviations: APL, abductor pollicis longus; DTML, deep transverse metacarpal ligament; EDM, extensor digiti minimi; FDP, flexor digitorum profundus.

finger. The slip of EDM is brought through the fourth and fifth metacarpal space into the volar wound. The tendon is then passed volar to the intermetacarpal ligament and brought back to the radial aspect of the small finger, where it is transferred to the lateral band or the radial aspect of the proximal phalanx as needed.

SUMMARY

Different patients have differing functional deficits after ulnar nerve palsy, ranging from aesthetic concerns to significant weakness in pinch. In dealing with the sequelae of late ulnar nerve palsy, each patient's needs should be carefully evaluated taking care to address the necessary issues. Multiple treatment options are available to restore function, and no single method can be applied to every case.[27] The authors' preferred methods for treatment of ulnar nerve palsy are presented in **Table 5**.

REFERENCES

1. Sachar K. Reconstruction for ulnar nerve palsy. In: Berger RA, Weiss AP, editors. Hand surgery. Philadelphia: Lippincott Williams & Wilkins; 2004. p. 979–90.
2. Schwarz RJ, Brandsma JW, Giurintano DJ. A review of the biomechanics of intrinsic replacement in ulnar palsy. J Hand Surg 2010;35B:94–102.
3. Taylor NL, Raj AD, Dick HM, et al. The correction of ulnar claw fingers: a follow-up study comparing the extensor-to-flexor with the palmaris longus 4 tailed tendon transfer in patients with leprosy. J Hand Surg 2004;29A:595–604.
4. Hollonshead WH. Anatomy for surgeons. 3rd edition. Philadelphia: Harper & Row; 1982.
5. Akboru IM, Solmaz I, Secer HI, et al. The surgical anatomy of the brachial plexus. Turk Neurosurg 2010;20:142–50.
6. Leinberry CF, Wehbe MA. Brachial plexus anatomy. Hand Clin 2004;20:1–5.
7. Sammer DM, Chung KC. Tendon transfers: part II. Transfers for ulnar nerve palsy and median nerve palsy. Plast Reconstr Surg 2009;124:212e–21e.
8. Posner MA. Compressive ulnar neuropathies at the elbow: I. Etiology and diagnosis. J Am Acad Orthop Surg 1998;6:282–8.
9. Leibovic SJ, Hastings H 2nd. Martin-Gruber revisited. J Hand Surg 1992;17A:47–53.
10. Kaplan EB, Spinner M. Normal and anomalous innervation patterns in the upper extremity. In: Omer GE Jr, Spinner M, editors. Management of peripheral nerve problems. Philadelphia: WB Saunders; 1980. p. 75–99.
11. Dumitru D, Walsh NE, Weber CF. Electrophysiologic study of the Riche-Cannieu anomaly. Electromyogr Clin Neurophysiol 1988;28:27–31.
12. Hastings H 2nd, Davidson S. Tendon transfers for ulnar nerve palsy: evaluation of results and practical treatment considerations. Hand Clin 1988;4: 167–78.
13. Vedamurthy M, IADVL Dematosurgery Task Force. Standard guidelines for the use of dermal fillers. Indian J Dermatol Venereol Leprol 2008;74:S23–7.

14. Butterwick KJ, Bevin AA, Iyer S. Fat transplantation using fresh versus frozen fat: a side-by-side two-hand comparison pilot study. Dermatol Surg 2006;32:640–4.

15. Markey AC, Glogau RG. Autologous fat grafting: comparison of techniques. Dermatol Surg 2000;26:1135–9.

16. Bertelli JA. Distal sensory nerve transfers in lower-type injuries of the brachial plexus. J Hand Surg 2012;37A:1194–9.

17. Brunelli GA. Sensory nerve transfers. J Hand Surg 2004;29B:557–62.

18. Mikhail IK. Bone block operation for claw hand. Surg Gynecol Obstet 1964;118:1077–9.

19. Zancolli EA. Claw hand caused by paralysis of the intrinsic muscles: a simple surgical procedure for its correction. J Bone Joint Surg Am 1957;39A:1076–80.

20. Bunnell S. Surgery of the intrinsic muscles of the hand other than those producing opposition of the thumb. J Bone Joint Surg Am 1942;24A:1–31.

21. Parkes A. Paralytic claw fingers: a graft tenodesis operation. Hand 1973;5:192–9.

22. Fowler SB. Extensor apparatus of the digits. J Bone Joint Surg 1949;31B:477.

23. Tsuge K. Tendon transfers in median and ulnar nerve paralysis. Hiroshima J Med Sci 1967;16:29–48.

24. Hastings H 2nd, McCollam SM. Flexor digitorum superficialis lasso tendon transfer in isolated ulnar nerve palsy: a functional evaluation. J Hand Surg 1994;19A:275–80.

25. Brown PW. Zancolli capsulorrhaphy for ulnar claw hand. J Bone Joint Surg Am 1970;52A:868–77.

26. Riordan DC. Intrinsic paralysis of the hand. Bull Hosp Jt Dis Orthop Inst 1984;44:435–41.

27. Riordan DC. Tendon transplantation in median nerve and ulnar nerve paralysis. J Bone Joint Surg Am 1953;35A:312.

28. Riordan DC. Rehabilitation and re-education in tendon transfers. Orthop Clin North Am 1974;5:445–9.

29. Stiles HJ, Forrester-Brown MF. Treatment of injuries of the spinal peripheral nerves. London: Henry Frowde and Hodder & Stoughton; 1922.

30. Brandsma JW, Ottenhoff-De Jonge MW. Flexor digitorum superficialis tendon transfer for intrinsic replacement. Long-term results and the effect on donor fingers. J Hand Surg 1992;17B:625–8.

31. Brand PW. Paralytic claw hand. J Bone Joint Surg 1958;40B:618.

32. Burkhalter WE. Restoration of power grip in ulnar nerve paralysis. Orthop Clin North Am 1974;5:289–303.

33. Enna CD, Riordan DC. The Fowler procedure for correction of the paralytic claw hand. Plast Reconstr Surg 1973;52:352–60.

34. Omer GE. Ulnar nerve palsy. In: Green DP, Hotchkiss WC, Pederson WC, editors. Green's operative hand surgery. 4th edition. New York: Churchill Livingstone; 1999. p. 1526–41.

35. Brand PW. Tendon grafting illustrated by a new operation for intrinsic paralysis of the fingers. J Bone Joint Surg 1961;43B:444–53.

36. Boyes JH. Bunnell's surgery of the hand. 5th edition. Philadelphia: Lippincott; 1970.

37. Smith RJ. Extensor carpi radialis brevis tendon transfer for thumb adduction—a study of power pinch. J Hand Surg 1983;8A:4–15.

38. Littler JW. Tendon transfers and arthrodesis in combined median and ulnar nerve palsies. J Bone Joint Surg Am 1949;31A:225–34.

39. North ER, Littler JW. Transferring the flexor superficialis tendon: technical considerations in the prevention of proximal interphalangeal joint instability. J Hand Surg 1980;5A:498–501.

40. Hamlin C, Littler JW. Restoration of power pinch. J Hand Surg 1980;5A:396–401.

41. Kozin SH, Bednar M. In vivo determination of available brachioradialis excursion during tetraplegia reconstruction. J Hand Surg 2001;26A:510–4.

42. Nevaiser RJ, Wilson JN, Gardner MM. Abductor pollicis longus transfer for replacement of first dorsal interosseous. J Hand Surg 1980;5A:53–7.

43. Burge P. Abducted little finger in low ulnar nerve palsy. J Hand Surg 1986;11B:234–6.

44. Blacker GJ, Lister GD, Kleinert HE. The abducted little finger in low ulnar nerve palsy. J Hand Surg 1976;1A:190–6.

45. Gonzalez MH, Gray T, Ortinau E, et al. The extensor tendons to the little finger: anatomic study. J Hand Surg 1995;20A:844–7.

46. Dellon AL. Extensor digiti minimi tendon transfer to correct abducted small finger in ulnar dysfunction. J Hand Surg 1991;16A:819–23.

Ulnar Neuropathy Following Distal Humerus Fracture Fixation

Alicia Worden, MD[a], Asif M. Ilyas, MD[b,c],*

KEYWORDS

- Ulnar nerve • Distal humerus fracture • In situ release • Transposition • Neuropathy

KEY POINTS

- Ulnar nerve injury can occur at the time of injury, during closed fracture manipulation, intraoperatively during fracture fixation, or during fracture healing.
- The authors recommend vigilance in ulnar nerve management during fixation of distal humerus fractures and routine disclosure to patients preoperatively concerning the high potential for postoperative ulnar neuropathy.
- Based on the best available evidence, the authors cannot recommend in situ release versus anterior transposition of the ulnar nerve intraoperatively. However, an anterior transposition in a subcutaneous fashion is recommended if increased tension on the ulnar nerve and/or direct hardware contact is noted intraoperatively following fracture fixation.

INTRODUCTION

Ulnar nerve dysfunction following distal humerus fractures is a well-recognized phenomenon. Its fixed anatomic position behind the medial epicondyle of the distal humerus predisposes the nerve to potential injury. Ulnar nerve injury can occur at the time of injury, during closed fracture manipulation, intraoperatively during open reduction internal fixation (ORIF), or during fracture healing and recovery.[1] During ORIF of distal humerus fractures, the ulnar nerve is routinely identified; however, intraoperative management varies widely. Some surgeons only perform in situ decompression,[2,3] others prefer routine transposition in all cases,[4–7] whereas others transpose the nerve only for specific indications related to preoperative nerve deficits, implant position, or to facilitate intraoperative nerve manipulation.[2,5,6,8–13] To better understand ulnar nerve dysfunction following operative management of distal humerus fractures, the authors evaluated the ulnar nerve function of patients treated with ORIF of distal humerus fractures over a 5-year period. We hypothesized that the (1) incidence of late ulnar nerve dysfunction following ORIF is higher than previously reported in the literature and (2) that the type of intraoperative nerve management does not significantly affect ulnar nerve dysfunction.

PATIENTS AND METHODS

After appropriate institutional review board approval was obtained, a retrospective chart review was performed of all patients aged 18 years and older that underwent ORIF for a distal humerus fracture, between 2004 and 2008 at a level I urban academic medical center. Patients were excluded if they had a preinjury history of ulnar nerve dysfunction. The minimum postoperative follow-up period was 6 months. A total of 24 patients were identified. Medical records and radiographs were reviewed in each case. Mechanism of injury, time to surgery, intraoperative

Disclosure: All named authors hereby declare that they have no conflicts of interest to disclose related to the topic of this article.
[a] Orthopaedic Surgery, Saint Louis University Hospital, 3635 Vista at Grand Blvd, St Louis, MO 63104, USA;
[b] Hand & Upper Extremity Surgery, Rothman Institute, 925 Chestnut Street, Philadelphia, PA 19107, USA;
[c] Orthopaedic Surgery, Thomas Jefferson University, 925 Chestnut Street, Philadelphia, PA 19107, USA
* Corresponding author.
E-mail address: asif.ilyas@rothmaninstitute.com

orthopedic.theclinics.com

fracture management, implants, intraoperative ulnar nerve management, perioperative ulnar nerve function, and late postoperative ulnar nerve function determined by McGowan[14] stages were recorded. Fractures were classified in accordance with the AO (Arbeitsgemeinschaft für Osteosynthesefragen) classification system[15] and the Gustilo and Anderson[16] classification system for open fractures. The patient's associated musculoskeletal injuries were also noted. Preoperative neurovascular examination of the affected upper extremity was documented in all cases except in three cases in which the patient was uncooperative or unresponsive.

Surgical approaches were divided into two types: either with or without olecranon osteotomy. During surgery, the ulnar nerve was routinely identified and protected in all cases. Ulnar nerve management was divided into three types: (1) in situ release, (2) subcutaneous anterior transposition, and (3) submuscular anterior transposition. Postoperatively, patients were treated with a posterior splint for approximately 2 weeks or less, followed by progressive range of motion. The classification for symptom occurrence was based on the time frames suggested by Shin and Ring[1] and included preoperative (injury induced), postoperative (within 2 weeks of operation), and subacute (occurrence after an asymptomatic 2 weeks of follow-up).

At final follow-up, McGowan[14] staging was performed to assess severity of ulnar nerve dysfunction. Grade I was defined as minimal lesions with no detectable motor weakness of the ulnar intrinsics and paresthesia in the ulnar nerve distribution with only slight blunting of sensation. Grade II was defined as intermediate lesions with weak interossei and muscle wasting as well as blunting of sensibility. Grade III was defined as a severe lesion with interossei paralysis and the marked hypoesthesia. This classification system is based on ulnar neuritis occurring after all causes with significant time for muscle atrophy. During follow-up of our patients, late complications and secondary procedures were also recorded.

RESULTS

A total of 31 patients had distal humerus fractures during the specified study period. However, 24 patients met the inclusion criteria. There were 9 women and 15 men. The average age was 46 (range 21–78). The average follow-up period was 13 months (range 6–26). The fractures were classified as seven AO type A (two A2 and five A3), two AO type B (all B1), and 15 AO type C (five C1, seven C2, and three C3). All patients underwent ORIF with plates and screws through a triceps-sparing approach, with 42% also requiring an olecranon

osteotomy. The mechanisms of injury included: fall on the outstretched arm (12, including four open-fracture cases), motor vehicle accidents (three total, including one open-fracture case), and gunshot fractures (eight total). A total of 20% (five out of 24) of the patients had preoperative neuropathy, with 12% (three out of 24) involving the radial nerve and only 8% (two out of 24) with ulnar neuropathies.

Intraoperative ulnar nerve management included 50% in situ release and 50% anterior transposition (one submuscular and 11 subcutaneous). At final follow-up, 38% (nine) patients had a persistent ulnar neuropathy. McGowan[14] stages included 56% stage 1 and 44% stage 2. There were no cases of McGowan[14] stage 3. Only two patients complained of preoperative ulnar paresthesias and both went on to have persistent ulnar neuropathy at final follow-up (one type 1 and one type 2). No patients with AO type B fractures developed late neuropathy, whereas three AO type A (all A3) and six AO type C (three C1, two C2, and one C1) did develop late neuropathy. Among the patients with persistent ulnar neuropathy at final follow-up, 44% (four) had undergone an in situ release and 56% (five) had undergone an anterior transposition. This difference was not statistically significant ($P>.05$). Among the patients with persistent ulnar neuropathy at final follow-up, 44% (four) had undergone ORIF without and 56% (five) had undergone ORIF with olecranon osteotomy. This was not statistically different ($P>.05$). In terms of implant, all fractures were treated with dual-column locking plates (one direct medial plate and one posterolateral plate) except for three cases treated with a single posterolateral locking plate. Late ulnar neuropathy was identified in 38% of dual-column plated fractures versus 33% of posterolateral-plated fractures. This was not statistically different ($P>.05$).

Among the McGowan[14] stage 1 patients, 40% had an olecranon osteotomy and 40% were AO type A versus 60% were AO type C fractures. Among the McGowan[14] stage 2 patients, 75% had an olecranon osteotomy and 25% were AO type A versus 75% were AO type C. All four McGowan[14] stage 2 and one McGowan[14] stage 1 patient ultimately required a second surgery involving removal of hardware and ulnar nerve neurolysis. All five patients had the second procedure performed at least 6 months after the index surgery. Among the cases without late ulnar neuropathy 20% (three out of 15) also underwent removal of hardware and joint release for painful hardware and/or elbow stiffness.

Discussion

We identified a 38% incidence of late ulnar neuropathy following ORIF of a distal humerus fracture, supporting our first hypothesis. This was most common in AO type C, followed by AO type A injuries. There were no cases of AO type B injuries resulting in late ulnar nerve dysfunction. The presence of a preoperative history of ulnar nerve paresthesias led to a 100% incidence of late symptoms. In no case was there a McGowan[14] stage 3 finding, but 56% were type 1 and 44% were type 2. All type 2 injuries ultimately required a second surgery to address ulnar nerve function. There was no statistical significance difference as to the development of late ulnar neuropathy and the surgical exposure, but there was a trend toward olecranon osteotomy. Supporting our second hypothesis, there was no statistical significance difference in general between the use of an in situ release versus transpositions and the development of late ulnar neuropathy, except for the single case using a submuscular transposition that ultimately led to late symptoms.

Ulnar Neuropathy Incidence

Nerve injuries, especially involving the ulnar nerve, are considered to be more often associated with severe fracture patterns. High-energy fractures dissipate their forces through the soft tissue and can also result in greater bone displacement. This can result in both direct and indirect nerve injury at the time of fracture. The incidence of ulnar neuropathy following distal humerus fracture fixation is variable. Occurrence presenting in the immediate postoperative period ranges from the low values of 0% to 6.6% to higher values of 10.1% to 21%.[2,4,5,9,11,12,14–20] Most of these reported postoperative neuropathies resolve with late ulnar neuropathy incidences ranging only from 0% to 3.3% but they have been documented at higher ranges of 11.7% to 16%.[2,4,5,11,14,15,17–20]

Helfet and Schmeling[8] retrospectively reviewed their experience with bicondylar intraarticular distal humerus fractures and identified, among other complications, a 7% incidence of late ulnar neuropathy but it was unclear from their series whether these were early or late neuropathies. More recently, Vazquez and colleagues[21] retrospectively examined 69 distal humerus fractures (both AO type A and C) without preoperative ulnar nerve symptoms to determine the incidence of late ulnar nerve dysfunction at a minimum of 12-months postoperatively. They identified an incidence of 10.1% immediately postoperatively and 16% at final follow-up. Also, using McGowan[14] staging, they identified that 57% were grade I and 43% were grade II and, similar to our series, no development of grade III stages. They also did not identify any specific risk factors for the development of late ulnar neuropathy. Moreover, Ruan and colleagues[3] retrospectively examined 117 consecutive AO type C distal humerus fractures at two centers to evaluate late ulnar nerve dysfunction and found that no patients without preoperative ulnar nerve symptoms developed late symptoms, whereas, among the 29 patients with preoperative ulnar nerve symptoms, there were 31% that continued to demonstrate late ulnar nerve symptoms.

Ulnar Nerve Management

There are inherent advantages and disadvantages to either releasing the ulnar nerve in situ or transposing it. In situ release affords surgical simplicity, decreased nerve handling, avoiding devascularization of the nerve, and iatrogenic traction injury. However, it maintains the nerve in close proximity to hardware in the cubital tunnel and tensioned around the medial epicondyle, in which case the native anatomy may also be altered. Transposition avoids contact of the nerve from fracture inflammation, callous formation, periarticular fibrosis, and soft tissue edema, as well as decreasing its tension along its path. However, transposition requires increased nerve handling, potential devascularization, traction injury, and late compressive neuropathy from inadequate decompression of soft tissue restraints.

Numerous recommendations have been made regarding when to transpose the ulnar nerve in distal humerus fracture management. An article reviewing distal humerus fractures from 1985 to 2003 advised transposition in those fractures with preoperative ulnar nerve symptoms, or when internal fixation requires extension over the medial epicondyle.[8] One investigator used indications of preoperative palsy, possible implant irritation, or intraoperative traction.[10,11] There continues to be no clear consensus as to when an ulnar nerve is transposed during surgery. The investigators' terminology in their decisions to transpose include "if hardware came to lie in the ulnar groove,"[9] "if during elbow flexion, ulnar nerve was noted to impinge on hardware,"[2] or "the ulnar nerve was mobilized if necessary to prevent iatrogenic damage."[20] Some investigators prefer to routinely transpose the ulnar nerve in all intrarticular distal humerus fractures,[4–6] whereas some investigators transpose without citing particular reasoning[18] and, in some cases, the investigators make no mention of their ulnar nerve management.[17,19]

The controversy is apparent when comparing studies analyzing similar fractures. The surgeons involved in the type C distal humerus fracture study by Athwal and colleagues[5] preferred to routinely anteriorly transpose the ulnar nerve in all cases with subcutaneous placement in 98%. Six patients

(19%) had preoperative ulnar nerve injuries. Similar to our transposition results, five patients (16%) had postoperative neuropathies (four ulnar and one radial sensory). The symptoms of three out of these five patients resolved at a mean of 4.5 months. The study did not specifically comment on the outcome of the preoperative neuropathic patients but did question whether the routine anterior transposition contributed to the increased incidence of postoperative ulnar neuropathy. However, another study by Luegmair and colleagues[18] with all type C fractures only transposed the nerve in two patients (12%). They reported only one (6%) of their 17 patients with preoperative ulnar symptoms and two (12%) postoperative ulnar neuropathies in patients without nerve transposition. Of note, the percentages of postoperative neuropathies is similar without transposition as reported by Luegmair and colleagues and with transposition, in both the results of our study and Athwal and colleagues' study.[5] Results, or without transposition as reported by Luegmair and colleagues.[18]

Other studies seem to favor anterior transposition of the ulnar nerve for both prevention and treatment of neuropathy. Gofton and colleagues[4] conducted another study analyzing type C fractures by assessed sensorimotor ulnar nerve outcomes with the 28-item Patient-Rated Ulnar Nerve Evaluation. Preoperatively, six patients (26%) had ulnar neuropathy. The investigators did not define the time frame for resolution but reported four of six patients' neuropathies resolving quickly. The other two preoperative neuropathies were categorized as subjective complaints after not finding any functional or objective deficits. Only one patient (4.3%) developed neuropathy after surgery, which could be classified as subacute or postoperative depending on the specific time-frame of symptom presentation. The investigators credit the low rate of objective ulnar neuropathy to routine transposition. Kinik and colleagues[6] also routinely transposed the ulnar nerve in their patients and had similar postoperative results. Three patients (6.5%) had ulnar neurapraxia caused initially by the fracture, whereas only two patients (4.3%) developed postoperative neuropathy. After transposition, the preoperative symptoms resolved and one of the two postoperative neuropathies improved during follow-up. One study by Wang and colleagues,[7] who performed anterior transposition during fixation of type C fractures, found none of their 20 patients developed postoperative or delayed ulnar neuropathies after adequate follow-up. Their results could be credited to small study group or other variables. No mention was made concerning the incidence of any preoperative symptoms.

In contrast, Robinson and colleagues[17] did not primarily transpose the ulnar nerve during treatment of distal humerus fractures—even with preoperative symptoms. Eight of their 320 patients (2.5%) had preoperative ulnar symptoms. One went on to have symptoms 3-months postinjury and treatment. Postoperatively, six patients (1.9%) developed ulnar neurapraxia and the investigators associated the palsy with surgical treatment of type C fractures. All but two palsies recovered postoperatively over 6 to 10 weeks. An additional study,[18] in which transposition was not routinely performed in all but two patients, also found good ulnar nerve recovery. Although it is not known which patients received the primary transpositions, it can be assumed that only the two postoperative neuropathic (11.7%) patients were not primarily transposed because they underwent additional ulnar nerve surgeries to treat their symptoms. Therefore, both studies had a small percentage of patients develop postoperative neuropathy without transposing the nerve.

In other studies, some investigators transposed the ulnar nerve based on simple criteria and produced favorable results. Two age-demographic studies of distal humerus fractures by Huang and colleagues[10,11] transposed the nerve with indications of preoperative palsy, possible implant irritation, and/or intraoperative traction of the nerve. In their study of elderly patients, they transposed the nerve based on their indications in 4.5%, 22.7%, and 4.5% of the patients.[10] In their larger study of all adult ages, they transposed the nerve in 5.0%, 12.5%, and 7.5% of patients based on their indications.[11] Overall, only one patient (5.3%) from their study of elderly patients and two patients (5%) from their study of adult patients developed a postoperative neuropathy. Ultimately, all patients with neuropathies resolved within 3 months. A group of surgeons in one study mobilized the ulnar nerve, if necessary, to prevent iatrogenic damage, although they did not give specific criteria.[20] Their rate of postoperative ulnar neurapraxia was 17%; however, all patients had resolved during follow-up.

The ulnar nerve can also be managed with in situ decompression. In a study by Russell and colleagues,[2] the surgeon initially performed what was described as an in-situ release of the ulnar nerve and would transpose the nerve only if during elbow flexion the nerve impinged on the hardware or subluxed. A total of seven patients (29%) had transpositions. Only one patient with transposition developed postoperative ulnar neuropathy, but symptoms resolved within 3 months. However, three patients (12.5%) without transposition postoperatively developed what the investigators called ulnar neuritis and attributed the results to the plating around the medial epicondyle.

A recent study by Ruan and colleagues[3] compared in situ decompression versus anterior subfascial (intramuscular) transposition of the ulnar nerve. The investigators chose a subfascial location because of its vascular bed as well as its decreased vulnerability to irritation and scarring when compared with submuscular alternatives. The 29 patients with preoperative ulnar symptoms (24.8%) were randomized to receive either ulnar nerve procedure. The Bishop rating system was used to classify ulnar nerve function. In the transposition group, 80% of the patients recovered completely, whereas the remaining 20% recovered partially. The in situ group had 57% of patients with complete recovery and 43% with only partial recovery. Furthermore, their rating system determined excellent and good results in 86.7% of the transposition group versus 57.1% of the in situ group. The results of this study advocate subfascial transposition over in situ release. Interestingly, the subfascial transposition was also performed on patients without preoperative symptoms and found no incidence of postoperative or delayed ulnar neuropathy.

SUMMARY

Many orthopedic surgeons have reported their findings in the treatment of distal humerus fractures. Earlier studies seem to have underreported ulnar neuropathy findings. The authors' data, as well as more recent available studies,[11,12] are in agreement that ulnar neuropathy is a common complication. In our patient cohort, there was an overall 38% incidence of persistent late ulnar neuropathy following fracture fixation, which included all patients with preoperative symptoms. This supports our first hypothesis that the incidence of late ulnar nerve dysfunction following ORIF is higher than previously reported in the literature. We also hypothesized that the type of intraoperative nerve management does not significantly affect ulnar nerve dysfunction. Among the patients with persistent ulnar neuropathy at final follow-up, 44% had undergone an in situ release and 56% had undergone an anterior transposition. This was not statistically different (P>.05). There was no statistically significant difference between an in situ release versus transposition and the development of late ulnar neuropathy, except for one case of submuscular transposition that ultimately led to late symptoms. Our study had several limitations. It was a single-center study. It was retrospective. The study sample size was small. Assessment of preoperative ulnar neuropathy was based on chart review. However, the study advantages included consistent surgical intervention and postoperative protocol, and standardized postoperative nerve assessment.

We recommend vigilance in ulnar nerve management during fixation of distal humerus fractures and routine disclosure to patients preoperatively concerning the high potential for postoperative ulnar neuropathy. Based on the best available evidence, we cannot recommend in situ release versus anterior transposition of the ulnar nerve intraoperatively. However, we would recommend an anterior transposition in a subcutaneous fashion if increased tension on the ulnar nerve and/or direct hardware contact is noted intraoperatively following fracture fixation. Moreover, we also believe that late compression of the ulnar nerve, if left within its native location within the cubital tunnel, may occur from fracture callus formation, surgical scar formation, and elbow stiffness resulting in loss of terminal extension, which is common following distal humerus fractures. If a transposition is undertaken, meticulous dissection of the nerve without its devascularization should be performed along with diligent removal of all potentially constricting soft tissue structures, including the arcade of Struthers, the intermuscular septum, Osborne's ligament, and the two heads of the flexor carpi ulnaris.

REFERENCES

1. Shin R, Ring D. The ulnar nerve in elbow trauma. J Bone Joint Surg Am 2007;89:1108–16.
2. Russell G, Jarrett C, Jones C, et al. Management of distal humerus fractures with minifragment fixation. J Orthop Trauma 2005;19:474–9.
3. Ruan H, Liu J, Fan C, et al. Incidence, management and prognosis of early ulnar nerve dysfunction in type C fractures of distal humerus. J Trauma 2009; 67(6):1397–401.
4. Gofton W, MacDermid J, Patterson S, et al. Functional outcome of AO type C distal humeral fractures. J Hand Surg 2003;28-A:294–308.
5. Athwal G, Hoxie S, Rispoli D, et al. Precontoured parallel plate fixation of AO/OTA type C distal humerus fractures. J Orthop Trauma 2009;23:575–80.
6. Kinik H, Atalar H, Mergen E. Management of distal humerus fractures in adults. Arch Orthop Trauma Surg 1999;119:467–9.
7. Wang K, Shih H, Hsu K, et al. Intercondylar fractures of the distal humerus: routine anterior subcutaneous transposition of the ulnar nerve in a posterior operative approach. J Trauma 2004;36(6):770–3.
8. Helfet D, Schmeling G. Bicondylar intrarticular fractures of the distal humerus in adults. Clin Orthop 1993;292:26–36.
9. Kundel K, Braun W, Wieberneit J, et al. Intraarticular distal humerus fractures: factors affecting functional outcome. Clin Orthop 1996;332:200–8.
10. Huang T, Chiu F, Chuang T, et al. The results of open reduction and internal fixation in elderly patients with

Carpal Tunnel Syndrome in Pregnancy

Meredith Osterman, MD[a], Asif M. Ilyas, MD[b],
Jonas L. Matzon, MD[b,*]

KEYWORDS

- Carpal tunnel syndrome • Median neuropathy • Pregnancy • Lactation

KEY POINTS

- Pregnancy is a risk factor for the development of median nerve compression or carpal tunnel syndrome.
- Pregnant women often experience nocturnal paresthesias that often can be effectively treated conservatively.
- If patients require surgical intervention for carpal tunnel syndrome, carpal tunnel release is considered a safe procedure that poses minimal risk to the mother or fetus.

INTRODUCTION

The physiology of pregnancy is complex and poses several challenges to physicians who are caring for the musculoskeletal health of pregnant women. Fluid changes, hormonal fluctuations, and increased weight gain all stress the muscular system and predispose patients to a plethora of orthopedic issues. One of the most common pregnancy-related ailments is carpal tunnel syndrome (CTS).

In the general population, the prevalence of CTS ranges from 0.7% to 9.2% among women and 0.4% to 2.1% among men.[1] These patients typically present with numbness in the median nerve distribution of the hand, wrist pain, nocturnal awakenings, decreased 2-point discrimination, and, in later stages, thenar muscle atrophy and weakness. In pregnant patients, CTS presents similarly. Most pregnant patients present with bilateral symptoms and most commonly in their third trimester, yet patients can present as early as the first few months of pregnancy and with unilateral symptoms.[2,3] The incidence of CTS in pregnancy has been reported to be as high as 62%; however, it varies widely in the literature.[4] For instance, the incidence of clinically diagnosed pregnancy-related CTS ranges from 31% to 62%, whereas the incidence of electrodiagnostically confirmed pregnancy-related CTS ranges from 7% to 43%.[5] Variations in study designs, specifically diagnostic criteria and methods, account for this wide distribution of incidence in the literature, and thus, the true incidence of pregnancy-related CTS is still unknown.

CAUSE OF PREGNANCY-RELATED CARPAL TUNNEL SYNDROME

Term pregnancy consists of 37 to 42 weeks of hormonal fluctuations, intravascular and extravascular fluid shifts, and musculoskeletal changes. Maternal blood volume may increase as much as 30% to 50% with a single pregnancy and up to 100% with twins or triplets.[6] The increased blood volume is a result of increases in both plasma and erythrocyte volume at a ratio of 2:1, yielding a dilutional anemia. Increased metabolism, increased

Disclosure: All named authors hereby declare that they have no conflicts of interest to disclose related to the topic of this article.
[a] Department of Orthopaedic Surgery, Thomas Jefferson University, 1015 Walnut Street Curtis Buliding, Suite 810, Philadelphia, PA 19107, USA; [b] Orthopaedic Surgery, Rothman Institute, Thomas Jefferson University, 925 Chestnut Street, Philadelphia, PA 19107, USA
* Corresponding author.
E-mail address: jonas.matzon@rothmaninstitute.com

heart rate, and increased stroke volume are coupled with a decrease in peripheral vascular resistance, and therefore the mean systemic blood pressure often is unchanged. Hormonal changes, such as increased levels of progesterone, rennin, and angiotensin, contribute to fluid retention, and this weight gain, coupled with the growth of the developing fetus, significantly taxes the musculoskeletal system. For instance, greater than 70% of pregnant women report back pain during the course of their pregnancy, making it the number one musculoskeletal condition in the peripartum period. The next most common musculoskeletal condition is CTS.[7,8]

The true cause of pregnancy-related CTS is unknown. It is thought to be multifactorial, with median nerve compression resulting as a consequence of normal physiologic changes of pregnancy. Increased fluid volume, uterine pressure on the inferior vena cava, progesterone-mediated hyperemia, and fluid retention lead to generalized edema during pregnancy. Swelling in the carpal tunnel can cause compression of the median nerve. Specifically, pregnant patients with hand swelling that prevents them from wearing their rings have an increased incidence of carpal tunnel symptoms.[2] In addition, patients who have gestational hypertension and preeclampsia have a higher incidence of CTS.[7] Although there is a strong correlation of generalized increased volume load (generalized edema) and development of CTS, there is little evidence to support a direct correlation between weight gain during pregnancy and CTS.[4,9]

It has also been shown that patients nursing their infants postpartum have increased development of CTS. These patients often have symptom relief with cessation of nursing.[2,7] However, the cause of this phenomenon is unknown. CTS related to nursing may be secondary to new repetitive hand positions, but it could also be the result of residual fluid and hormonal changes associated with pregnancy. Lactating patients who develop CTS tend not to have preeclampsia or generalized edema during pregnancy.[4] These patients also have a slower time course to symptom resolution, compared with resolution of carpal tunnel symptoms that begin during pregnancy.[4] The literature has not addressed the causation between median nerve compression and lactation, yet a relationship has been well observed.

There is a known association between altered glucose metabolism, such as that in diabetes, and the development of CTS. Impaired fasting glucose levels and increased insulin resistance are independent risk factors for the development of CTS and, more specifically, for the development of bilateral disease.[10–12] Pregnant women undergo alterations in glucose metabolism, including increased fasting insulin levels, increased hepatic glucose production, and decreased insulin sensitivity, to compensate for the increased metabolic demands of the mother and fetus.[10] These endocrine adaptations of pregnancy would be expected to contribute to the development of CTS via a similar mechanism as that in diabetic patients.[11] However, diabetes has not been proved to be a risk factor for the development of pregnancy-related CTS.[13]

Finally, pregnancy may predispose women to nerve hypersensitivity. A study in dogs from Japan has shown that pregnant dogs have abnormal nerve susceptibility to pressure.[14] In humans, a recent study evaluated 2 groups of age-matched women (1 group of pregnant women and 1 group of nonpregnant women) with the use of electrodiagnostic testing. Neither group had any hand symptoms or any clinical indication of median nerve pathologic conditions. However, on electrodiagnostic testing, 11% of the asymptomatic pregnant women had median nerve impairment compared with the asymptomatic nonpregnant group, implying a subclinical median neuropathy associated with pregnancy. Of note, 4 of the asymptomatic pregnant patients with subclinical median nerve compression developed symptoms of CTS later in their pregnancy.[15] Perhaps the hormonal changes and increased volume of pregnancy provide a double-hit phenomenon on an overly susceptible median nerve. Can an increase in the volume within the carpal tunnel that would otherwise be insignificant cause the compression of a hypersensitive nerve?

EVALUATION OF THE PREGNANT PATIENT

Evaluating the pregnant patient with CTS is no different than evaluating any new patient presenting with hand paraesthesias. A thorough history and physical examination are warranted. The history should elucidate the duration, quality, and consistency of symptoms. Specifically, it is necessary to understand the distribution of the numbness and whether the symptoms are constant or intermittent. For pregnant patients, it is imperative to also inquire about gestational age, weight gain, nulliparity, excessive edema, previous pregnancy-related CTS, and any current complications of pregnancy, such as preeclampsia and/or gestational (pregnancy-induced) hypertension.

The classic presentation of CTS is numbness and pain in the palmar thumb, index finger, long finger, and radial half of the ring finger. Patients may complain of aching in the thenar eminence, weakness in thumb opposition, and thenar atrophy.

Difficulties with activities such as buttoning shirts, writing, combing hair, and driving a car are common complaints. Symptoms are frequently exacerbated by repetitive hand motion and/or sleep. Furthermore, greater than 50% of pregnant patients report symptom exacerbation during the night.[7] Compared with patients with idiopathic CTS, pregnant patients with CTS report significantly more pain and numbness.[16]

When obtaining the history, it is important to discern the onset of symptoms. Pregnant patients presenting in their first 2 trimesters characteristically have more acute, rapidly progressing symptoms for which conservative treatment often fails. Electrodiagnostic testing of these patients can confirm acute median nerve lesions with motor and/or sensory conduction blocks at the wrist that may ultimately require surgical intervention.[17] Seror described one patient who developed the rapid onset of conduction delays only 5 days after the onset of her symptoms.[16] In contrast, when CTS occurs during the third trimester, it often has a slower onset of symptoms that frequently responds well to conservative treatment and usually resolves postdelivery.

During the physical examination, detailed attention should focus on sensory deficits, 2-point discrimination, muscle strength, and thenar atrophy. Provocative examination maneuvers that are useful in the diagnosis of CTS include Phalen's test, reverse Phalen's test, Tinel's test, and Durkin's compression test. The onset of numbness and tingling in the distribution of the median nerve during any of these maneuvers is a positive test. These maneuvers aid in making a clinical diagnosis but none have 100% sensitivity. For example, the sensitivity for Tinel's test ranges from 45% to 75%, and that for Phalen's test ranges from 49% to 89%.[18] More recently, Cheng and colleagues reported a new provocative test called the scratch collapse test. It involves the clinician lightly scratching over the median nerve while the patient performs resisted shoulder external rotation. The test is positive if the patient demonstrates momentary loss of external resistance after scratching over the median nerve.[18] This test is unique in that it does not rely on subjective patient response, like the other provocative tests described. It has been found to have 64% sensitivity in diagnosing CTS and a higher negative predictive value compared with Tinel's and Phalen's tests.

DIAGNOSTIC TESTING OF THE PREGNANT PATIENT

Although CTS is a clinical diagnosis, electrodiagnostic studies can be helpful in confirming the diagnosis and clarifying the severity of the disease. Nerve conduction studies and electromyography are used to evaluate the health of a nerve axon, the associated myelin, and the innervation of specific muscles. As nerves are compressed, demyelination occurs, which slows conduction velocity of the nerve across the compressed site. As compression continues, axonal loss results in decreased recruitment of motor unit potentials. Both of these values are evident on nerve conduction studies. As muscles become denervated, electromyography will show fibrillations and decreased recruitment of motor unit potentials.

Not only are electrodiagnostic studies useful in staging the degree of nerve compression and in assessing nerve damage but they also have prognostic value. These tests can allow for more reliable patient and surgeon postoperative expectations. For example, if the nerve is severely compressed and the thenar muscles show fibrillations and denervation, the patient should be counseled that surgical intervention may not completely alleviate the symptoms but may merely halt the progression of nerve damage. These studies can also aid in differentiating CTS from other peripheral nerve problems, such as cervical radiculopathy, brachial plexopathy, or more proximal median nerve compression.

The indication for electrodiagnostic studies in a pregnant patient is not clearly defined. For the general population, the American Academy of Orthopaedic Surgeons has produced clinical practice guidelines on the diagnosis of CTS.[19] These guidelines, which were adopted in May 2007, gave the highest recommendation (fair, levels II and III) to obtain electrodiagnostic tests if clinical and/or provocative tests are positive and surgical management is being considered. Given that surgery is not frequently considered during pregnancy and that symptoms frequently abate after delivery, electrodiagnostic testing can often be avoided. However, severe symptoms such as constant numbness, thenar weakness, and/or thenar atrophy require prompt attention. To fully understand the severity of the median nerve compression and to avoid the potential of irreversible changes, physicians may consider ordering nerve conduction and electrodiagnostic studies.

Interpreting electrodiagnostic studies in pregnant patients is the same as for the general population. For median nerve compression, both sensory and distal motor nerve latency is evaluated. Sensory latency is more sensitive and is the earliest indicator of CTS on electrodiagnostic testing. If the sensory latency is absent, motor latency can be used. For accurate diagnosis, it is necessary to have radial or ulnar sensory latencies of the same hand for comparison. A sensory latency of greater than 3.5 ms or abnormal comparative tests is diagnostic of CTS. Patients with severe disease will also have prolonged distal motor latency (usually >4 ms) and/or absent sensory/motor latency and absent muscle action potentials. However, the correlation between patient symptoms and findings on electrodiagnostic testing is not well established.[20]

Studies have compared electrodiagnostic findings in pregnant and nonpregnant patients with CTS. Seror showed that mean conduction velocity impairment was equivocal in pregnant and nonpregnant patients with CTS; however; the pregnant patients developed latency within 3 months compared with 41 months in the nonpregnant patients.[16] Weimer and colleagues[21] followed a pregnant patient presenting with signs of CTS using electrodiagnostic testing and clinical examinations. A normal study conducted 1 year before pregnancy was used as a control. Serial nerve conduction studies were performed weekly on this patient, beginning at 22 weeks of gestation (2 weeks after the onset of symptoms) through delivery, then at 3 separate time points postpartum. The patient had decline of all measurements (sensory nerve action potential [SNAP], conduction velocity [CV], distal motor latency [DML], amplitude) compared with the control values at week 22, which coincided with symptom onset. At week 24, treatment was initiated with bilateral wrist splints and salt reduction. Following the onset of treatment, amplitude showed steady, progressive improvement. However, latency measurements declined until week 27 and then showed improvement. By 20 weeks postpartum, the electrodiagnostic values returned to baseline (similar to the values seen at 1 year prepregnancy). This case illustrates the close correlation between symptom onset and electrodiagnostic findings. Furthermore, it demonstrates that pregnancy-related CTS does not completely resolve with delivery.

COURSE OF PREGNANCY-RELATED CARPAL TUNNEL SYNDROME

Although the symptoms are similar, the course of CTS is different in pregnant patients than in the standard population. Although the cause of CTS is not clear, it is often believed to be secondary to overuse activities (eg, flexor tendon tenosynovitis and inflammation), metabolic changes (eg, diabetes), or anatomic variants (eg, a lumbrical muscle or a mass within the canal). Therefore, an intervention such as behavior modification, local anti-inflammatory medications, glucose control, or

surgical decompression of the carpal tunnel is usually necessary to alleviate symptoms. In contrast, pregnancy-related CTS begins in pregnancy, which implies that the cause is solely pregnancy-related changes. It is naturally assumed that once the pregnancy has ended, the symptoms will resolve. However, the literature shows a large variation in the course of the disease. Wand reported that 95% of pregnant patients with CTS had resolution of their symptoms within 2 weeks of delivery and the remainder within 1 month.[2] Other studies have shown that as many as 50% of patients have CTS symptoms at 1 year after delivery of their child.[22] Many of these patients are breastfeeding, which may prolong recovery, but it has been reported that up to 50% of patients have symptoms as long as 3 years after delivery, long after the cessation of nursing.[7] Even without clinical symptoms, some of these patients have objective findings, such as positive Phalen's sign, motor weakness of the abductor pollicis brevis, and sensory loss in the median nerve distribution, after delivery.[3]

TREATMENT OPTIONS FOR PREGNANCY-RELATED CARPAL TUNNEL SYNDROME

Treatment of CTS in a pregnant patient is similar to that in the general population. Conservative treatment is the initial route with nighttime neutral wrist splints and local corticosteroid injections into the carpal tunnel. Surgical decompression is often warranted after failure of conservative treatment or with significant nerve compression seen on electrodiagnostic testing. According to the American Academy of Orthopaedic Surgeons' clinical practice guidelines on the treatment of CTS, there is no specific evidence to provide treatment recommendations when CTS is associated with pregnancy.[19]

In the general population, CTS is often a progressive process in which conservative measures will likely fail during a period of time and patients ultimately will need surgical intervention. In contrast, up to 85% of cases of pregnancy-related CTS resolve within 2 to 4 weeks of delivery.[23] Therefore, the goal is to keep patients comfortable as they progress through their pregnancy and to use surgical decompression for patients not responding to conservative care or those with significant nerve compression on electrodiagnostic studies.[24] With conservative care, patients with pregnancy-related CTS have a 3 to 4 times greater probability of improving compared with nonpregnant patients with CTS.[24] In fact, 82% of pregnant patients have good relief of symptoms using nighttime splints alone.[23]

Local corticosteroid injections into the carpal tunnel have good clinical outcomes in the general and pregnant population, with up to 50% of patients having sustained improvement of symptoms for longer than 15 months. When steroid injections were compared with placebo injections at 1 month, the patients with steroid injections showed greater improvement.[25] In a recent study, visual pain scores and electrodiagnostic studies were performed on symptomatic pregnant women both before and 3 weeks after an injection with dexamethasone and 1% lidocaine. Eighty percent of the patients reported a significant decrease in symptoms, and the diagnostic tests demonstrated statistically significant decreases in sensory nerve conduction velocity, distal motor latency, and distal sensory latency.[26] However, steroid injections are most beneficial in patients with mild to moderate carpal tunnel disease (sensory latency >3.5 ms and distal motor latency >4.2 ms, both <6 ms).[26] Furthermore, some patients are concerned about the effects of steroid injections on the health of their unborn child. To date, no study has examined this question specifically; however, steroids are known to aid in surfactant production and lung tissues development in premature babies, so intuitively, it would seem that a local injection into the carpal tunnel would have little significance for the fetus.[27]

When conservative management fails or patients demonstrate significant electrodiagnostic changes, surgical release of the transverse carpal ligament is recommended. There is minimal risk to mother or child when the procedure is done under local anesthetic and using a tourniquet.[28] In fact, 98% of pregnant patients report an excellent result after surgical decompression.[28] Complications of CTS are not unique to the pregnant patient and include wound infection, inadequate ligament release, fibrosis/scarring of the flexor tendons, and injury to the median nerve or its branches.[29]

SUMMARY

The issue of CTS in pregnant and lactating women remains a clinical mystery. Why is it that pregnant patients have glucose intolerance similar to diabetic patients, yet a clear association between patients with gestational diabetes and CTS does not exist? Why is it that some pregnant patients have complete resolution of their symptoms after delivery, whereas others remain symptomatic for months?

The true cause of pregnancy-related CTS may never be defined. What is important to acknowledge is that pregnancy is a risk factor for the development of median nerve compression and that

often these patients present with symptoms that may warrant the implementation of conservative or operative intervention. Most pregnant patients who develop CTS will have complete resolution after delivery. For the few who present with significant clinical findings suggesting severe nerve compression, the physician should consider obtaining electrodiagnostic studies early to help quantify the degree of nerve compression. In addition, it is important to recognize that some of these patients may not get better after delivery and may require continued postpartum conservative care or surgical treatment.

REFERENCES

1. Andersen JH, Thomsen JF, Overgaard E, et al. Computer use and carpal tunnel syndrome: a 1-year follow-up study. JAMA 2003;289(22):2963–9.
2. Wand JS. Carpal tunnel syndrome in pregnancy and lacation. J Hand Surg Br 1990;15(1):93–5.
3. Melvin JL, Burneett CN, Johnson EW. Median nerve conduction in pregnancy. Arch Phys Med Rehabil 1969;50:75–80.
4. Padua L, Aprile I, Caliandro P, et al, Italian Carpal Tunnel Study Group. Symptoms and neurophysiological picture of carpal tunnel syndrome in pregnancy. Clin Neurophysiol 2001;112:1946–51.
5. Padua L, Di Pasquale A, Pazzaglia C, et al. Systematic review of pregnancy-related carpal tunnel syndrome. Muscle Nerve 2010;42:697–703.
6. Foley M. Materlan cardiovascular and hemodynamic adaptations to pregnancy. UpToDate; 2010.
7. Heckman JD, Sassard R. Musculoskeletal considerations in pregnancy. J Bone Joint Surg Am 1994;76: 1720–30.
8. Voitk AL, Mueller JC, Farlinger DE, et al. Carpal tunnel syndrome in pregnancy. Can Med Assn J 1983;128:277–81.
9. Stolp-Smith KA, Pascoe MK, Ogburn PL Jr. Carpal tunnel syndrome in pregnancy: frequency, severity, and prognosis. Arch Phys Med Rehabil 1998;79: 1285–7.
10. Becker J, Nora D, Gomes I, et al. An evaluation of gender, obesity, age and diabetes mellitus as risk factors for carpal tunnel syndrome. Clin Neurophysiol 2002;113(9):1429–34.
11. Plastino M, Fava A, Carmela C, et al. Insulin resistance increases risk of carpal tunnel syndrome: a case-control study. J Peripher Nerv Syst 2011; 16(3):186–90.
12. Lain K, Catalano P. Metabolic changes in pregnancy. Clin Obstet Gynecol 2007;50(4):934–48.
13. Turgut F, Cetinsahinahin M, Turgut M, et al. The management of carpal tunnel syndrome in pregnancy. J Clin Neurosci 2001;8:332–4.

14. Takayama S. An experimental study on compression neuropathy. The vulnerability of the peripheral nerve associated with pregnancy. Nihon Seikeigeka Gakkai Zasshi 1990;64:485–99 [in Japanese].

15. Baumann F, Karlikaya G, Yuksel G, et al. The subclinical incidence of CTS in pregnancy: assessment of median nerve impairment in asymptomatic pregnant women. Neurol Neurophysiol Neurosci 2007;3.

16. Seror P. Pregnancy-related carpal tunnel syndrome. J Hand Surg Br 1998;23(1):98–101.

17. Stahl S, Blumenfeld Z, Yarnitsky D. Carpal tunnel syndrome in pregnancy: indications for early surgery. J Neurol Sci 1996;136:182–4.

18. Cheng C, Mackinnon-Patterson B, Beck J, et al. Scratch collapse test for evaluation of carpal and cubital tunnel syndrome. J Hand Surg Am 2008;33:1518–24.

19. Keith MW, Masear V, Chung KC, et al. AAOS clinical practice guidelines on treatment of carpal tunnel syndrome. J Bone Joint Surg Am 2010;92:218–9.

20. Werner R, Andary M. Electrodiagnostic evaluation of carpal tunnel syndrome. Muscle Nerve 2011;44:597–607.

21. Weimer L, Yin J, Lovelace RE, et al. Serial studies of carpal tunnel syndrome during and after pregnancy. Muscle Nerve 2002;25:914–7.

22. Sax T, Rosenbaum R. Neuromuscular disorders in pregnancy. Muscle Nerve 2006;34:559–71.

23. Ekman-Ordeberg G, Salgeback S, Ordeberg G. Carpal tunnel syndrome in pregnancy. A prospective study. Acta Obstet Gynecol Scand 1987;66:233–5.

24. Mondelli M, Rossi S, Monti E, et al. Prospective study of positive factors for improvement of carpal tunnel syndrome in pregnant women. Muscle Nerve 2007;36(6):778–83.

25. Visser L, Ngo Q, Groeneweg S, et al. Long term effect of local corticosteroid injection for carpal tunnel syndrome: a relation with electrodiagnostic severity. Clin Neurophysiol 2012;123(4):838–41.

26. Moghtaderi AR, Mohgtaderi N, Loghmani A. Evaluating the effectiveness of local dexamethasone injection in pregnant women with carpal tunnel syndrome. J Res Med Sci 2011;16(5):687–90.

27. Morgan M, Goldenber R, Schulkin J. Obstetrician-gynecologists screening and management of preterm birth. Obstet Gynecol 2008;112:35–41.

28. Assmus H, Hshemi B. Surgical treatment of carpal tunnel syndrome in pregnancy: results from 31 cases. Nervenarzt 2000;71:470–3.

29. Hunt TR, Osterman AL. Complications of the treatment of carpal tunnel syndrome. Hand Clin 1974;10:63–71.

Carpal Tunnel Syndrome After Distal Radius Fracture

Genghis E. Niver, MD, Asif M. Ilyas, MD*

KEYWORDS

- Carpal tunnel syndrome • Median neuropathy • Distal radius fracture • Wrist fracture

KEY POINTS

- The treating surgeon should be vigilant in noticing the signs and symptoms of carpal tunnel syndrome.
- If early carpal tunnel syndrome findings are noted during distal radius fracture management, all potential causes should be evaluated, including prominent volar cortical fragments causing direct compression of the median nerve, inadequate fracture reduction, and iatrogenic causes such as prominently placed hardware.
- Delayed carpal tunnel syndrome presenting after a distal radius fracture has healed is best managed in standard fashion.

BACKGROUND

Both carpal tunnel syndrome (CTS) and distal radius fractures are among the most common diagnoses of conditions treated by hand surgeons and orthopedic surgeons. However, their relationship to each other is poorly understood. Distal radius fractures are the most common fractures seen in the emergency department, with an incidence of more than 640,000 per year in the United States.[1–3] A bimodal distribution of distal radius fractures is seen, with one peak representing predominantly young male patients sustaining high-energy injuries and another peak representing predominantly elderly female patients sustaining low-energy fragility fractures.[4,5] Common complications that occur following distal radius fractures include arthrosis, malunion, nonunion, tendon rupture, chronic regional pain syndrome (CRPS), ulnar impaction, loss of rotation, finger stiffness, and, rarely, compartment syndrome.[6] Another known complication of distal radius fractures is median nerve compression at the wrist, or CTS. A review of 565 patients revealed immediate or delayed CTS as the most common complication with distal radius fracture.[7] The time for onset of CTS after distal radius fracture can vary from a few hours to many years.[8] CTS can be classified as idiopathic (or primary), secondary, and acute. Idiopathic (or primary) CTS is the most common form and results in a multifactorial manner presenting most commonly in the fourth to fifth decade resulting in progressive median nerve paraesthesias that is worsened with activity and flexed positioning of the wrist. Idiopathic CTS is also the most common complaint of the hand. Secondary CTS occurs from anatomic changes to the carpal tunnel, space-occupying lesions, and inflammatory conditions resulting in increased pressure within the carpal tunnel. Acute CTS is progressive in nature, develops rapidly, and consists of painful paraesthesias in the median nerve distribution of the hand.

Disclosure: All named authors hereby declare that they have no conflicts of interest to disclose related to the topic of this article.

Hand and Upper Extremity Surgery, Rothman Institute, Thomas Jefferson University, 925 Chestnut Street, Philadelphia, PA 19107, USA

* Corresponding author.
E-mail address: asif.ilyas@rothmaninstitute.com

orthopedic.theclinics.com

Acute CTS has been reported to occur in 5.4% to 8.6% of all distal radius fractures.[7,9–11] Secondary CTS can occur months to years after a distal radius fracture. This presentation is usually associated with a malunion or residual displacement of the distal radius fragment, chronic edema of the tenosynovium, prolonged immobilization in the Cotton-Loder position, and enlarging callus.[7,10,12–19] The incidence of delayed CTS after a distal radius fracture is estimated to be 0.5% to 22%.[14,20–24]

DIAGNOSIS

The major complaints with CTS are numbness and paraesthesias in the median nerve distribution of the hand and weakness in thumb opposition. Physical examination will note possible paraesthesias in the thumb, index and middle fingers, and radial half of the ring fingers. Semmes-Weinstein monofilament testing is the most sensitive in detecting sensory threshold changes in CTS.[25] Symptoms may be brought on with prolonged wrist flexion (Phalen's test) or direct compression of the median nerve at the carpal tunnel (Durkan's test). Strength testing may identify weakness in resisted thumb abduction and atrophy of the thenar musculature. In the setting of a distal radius fracture, CTS symptoms may be worsened with progressive deformity and swelling (**Fig. 1**).

PATHOPHYSIOLOGY

Dyer and colleagues[11] thought that "acute CTS should be distinguished from median nerve dysfunction due to deformity or contusion: the former usually develops slowly over hours to days and progressively worsens, whereas the latter is present at the time of injury, often improves after manipulative reduction, and tends to improve within days to weeks." The potential effects of unrecognized or untreated CTS are permanent dysfunction of the median nerve and possibly CRPS.[25–27] Therefore, the clinician must act expeditiously if CTS symptoms arise.

Acute Canal Pressure Changes

Many authors have analyzed and explored the possible mechanisms of the development of CTS after a distal radius fracture. Increased compartment pressures are a major cause of acute CTS after a distal radius fracture. Kongsholm and Olerud[28] measured carpal canal pressures in patients with a distal radius fracture before injection with a local anesthetic and compared this group to a control group of healthy volunteers.

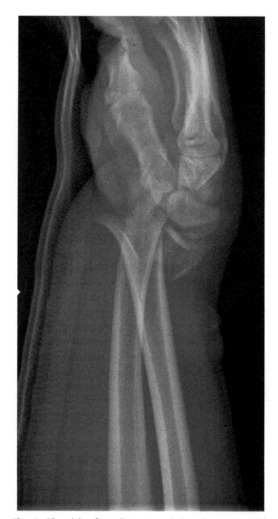

Fig. 1. The risk of median nerve injury increases with progressive deformity and fracture displacement. Note the extent of deformity following complete dorsal displacement of the distal radius fracture. This patient was originally splinted in this displaced position and presented with progressive median nerve paraesthesias. However, following provisional fracture reduction, the paraesthesias resolved.

They concluded that the injection of a local anesthetic at the time of manual reduction increased the carpal canal pressure, as did volar flexion of the wrist. Similarly, Gelberman and colleagues[29] measured carpal canal pressures in patients with a distal radius fracture at various positions of flexion or extension. They found that 10 (45%) of 23 fractured wrists had carpal canal pressures greater than 40 mm Hg in 40° of flexion. In addition to position, increased carpal canal pressure may be due directly to the hematoma resulting from a distal radius fracture, which may extravasate into the carpal tunnel.[8,17]

Alteration in Carpal Tunnel Anatomy

Beyond canal pressure changes in the acute period, chronic changes to the carpal tunnel anatomy following a distal radius fracture may also result in the development of CTS. Excessive volar callus formation can cause direct nerve compression during the healing phase of a distal radius fracture.[7,30] This would most likely present with delayed symptoms as callus forms over weeks. Lynch and Lipscomb described the potential contribution of the inflammation of flexor tendon tenosynovitis to the development of CTS following a distal radius fracture.[31] Furthermore, Lynch and Lipscomb postulated that another cause of CTS following a distal radius fracture is a resulting malunion leading to anatomic alterations within the carpal tunnel, resulting in decreased space and/or a new abnormal course for the median nerve to traverse.

Direct Median Nerve Injury

Other studies have proposed that direct trauma to the median nerve at the time of injury can be a cause of CTS after a distal radius fracture. Median nerve injury has been reported with volar cortical fragments directly injuring the median nerve after a fracture (**Fig. 2**).[32–34] The authors

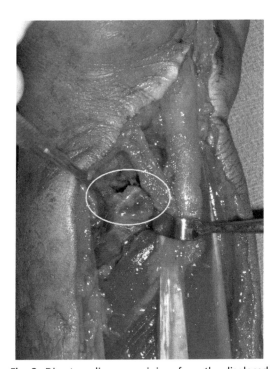

Fig. 2. Direct median nerve injury from the displaced volar cortical fragment is impinging on the median nerve. This patient presented with acute CTS requiring urgent decompression and fracture reduction.

recommended early carpal tunnel release (CTR) with removal or reduction of the volar fragment. A displaced volar fracture fragment has also been implicated in tardy median nerve palsy.[7,35–37] Such cases may present months after the injury as a result of direct pressure on the median nerve and/or alterations of the anatomy within the carpal tunnel.

WHAT IS THE EVIDENCE?

Numerous studies have speculated as to the causes of median nerve injury and median nerve compression after a distal radius fracture.[11,38–42] In a retrospective case-control study by Dyer and colleagues[11] reviewed orthopedic trauma and billing databases for all surgically treated fractures of the distal radius in a 5-year period at 2 level 1 trauma centers. After exclusion criteria were accounted for, the total cohort between the 2 centers included 50 patients. The proposed risk factors for acute CTS included injury mechanism (low-energy, high-energy, and crush injuries), open fracture, ipsilateral wrist injury, ipsilateral upper extremity injury, and multiorgan system injuries. The authors concluded that ipsilateral upper extremity trauma (with hand fractures excluded) and translation of the fracture fragments were significant predictors of acute CTS. Weaknesses of the study include its retrospective nature, selection bias that may be present at level 1 trauma centers, and the large percentage of patients excluded as a result of missing or inadequate pre-reduction radiographs.

Itsubo and colleagues[38] also performed a retrospective study in which they evaluated onset patterns and causes of CTS after a distal radius fracture. In their review, treatment was closed reduction and cast immobilization in 75 wrists, external fixation in 9 wrists, closed reduction and percutaneous pinning in 7 wrists, open reduction and internal fixation in 10 wrists, and corrective radius osteotomy after closed reduction and cast immobilization in 4 wrists. Treatments for CTS included CTR in 68 wrists, CTR with corrective radial osteotomy in 5 wrists, corrective radial osteotomy alone in 2 wrists, and conservative treatment only (steroid injection or splinting) in 30 wrists. Based on the results of the review, the authors noted that patients in the acute-onset group were significantly younger and had a higher proportion of male patients compared with the other 2 onset groups. In addition, the incidence of a high-energy injury was significantly higher in the acute-onset group than in the other 2 onset groups. Based on radiographic classification, the authors also concluded that the incidence of AO type C fractures was significantly higher in the acute-onset group than in the other 2 onset groups.

Unlike the study by Itsubo and colleagues, Bienek and colleagues[39] prospectively followed the outcomes of 60 patients who presented with distal radius fractures and developed peripheral nerve compression during a 5-year period. Of the 60 patients in the study, 12 patients had symptoms of CTS and the diagnosis was confirmed electrodiagnostically. Those 12 patients had significantly worse subjective scores than the 48 patients without CTS. The authors were not able to demonstrate a correlation between the occurrence of CTS and the fracture type according to the AO classification. In addition, correlation was not observed between radiographic end results (radial inclination, volar tilt, and radial shortening) and the occurrence of CTS.

Many authors have attempted to study the relationship between compartment pressure in the carpal tunnel and acute median neuropathy after a distal radius fracture. Dresing and colleagues[41] measured compartment pressures in a prospective controlled study in 56 patients. Measurements were taken at initial presentation, immediately before and after reduction, and 1, 2, 4, 12, and 24 hours after reduction. Sixteen patients underwent primary surgery and 4 patients had secondary surgery. All wrists were positioned in 25° of flexion and 20° of ulnar deviation after reduction. These fractured wrists were all casted and the respective casts were all split. All fractures were also grouped into the appropriate AO classification for distal radius fractures. Three measurements were taken using an intracompartmental pressure monitor system, 5 minutes after insertion of the catheter. The highest peak pressure (mean of 44.3 mm Hg) was seen at the time of reduction and a second peak occurred 4 hours after reduction (mean 37.0 mm Hg). The highest pressure was observed immediately after reduction before splitting of the cast. A sudden drop in pressure was instantaneously observed after splitting and loosening of the cast. Four patients eventually developed CRPS. Three of these patients had significantly elevated carpal pressures during reduction or afterward. One female patient had pressures exceeding 80 mm Hg and required median nerve decompression along with open reduction and internal fixation. The authors were also able to conclude that AO A2-type fractures had a significantly lower carpal tunnel pressure at the time of admission (average 16.1 mm Hg) compared with A3-type (average 25.5 mm Hg) and C2-type (average 27.7 mm Hg; $P = .01$) fractures.

Similarly, Fuller and colleagues[42] measured carpal tunnel pressures in 10 patients who underwent open reduction and internal fixation of a distal radius fracture through a volar approach during a 7-month period. Surgery was performed using a volar approach, with a slit catheter inserted under direct visualization on the radial aspect of the median nerve in the carpal canal. During layered closure of the wound, the catheter was brought out through the proximal end of the surgical wound and a volar plaster splint was applied. Carpal canal pressures were measured every 2 hours during the first 24 hours postoperatively, when the catheter was removed. The maximum recorded carpal canal pressure was 65 mm Hg in the only patient with fracture blisters. That patient had a trending decrease in pressures down to 31 mm Hg by the end of the study period. In addition, that patient never had signs of acute CTS. Of note, the same patient had a history of systemic hypertension, which may have offered a protective mechanism during his recovery. The general trend of the carpal canal pressures was a decrease during the 24 hours of monitoring. Most patients had carpal canal pressures less than the safe threshold pressure of 40 to 50 mm Hg proposed by Gelberman and colleagues.[29] Based on their findings, Fuller and colleagues concluded that "routine prophylactic carpal tunnel release is not recommended after volar plating of distal radius fractures."[42]

TREATMENT

The unintended consequences of unrecognized or untreated CTS can be devastating. Many nonsurgical and surgical options have been described in the literature aiming at preventing and treating CTS after a distal radius fracture. In 2009, the American Academy of Orthopaedic Surgeons (AAOS) published treatment guidelines for adult distal radius fractures.[43–46] With regard to operative intervention for CTS after a distal radius fracture, the AAOS treatment guidelines did not recommend for or against performing nerve decompression when nerve dysfunction persists after reduction,[43] because the inconclusive evidence in the literature could not provide enough support based on qualified studies.

Although the AAOS treatment guidelines for adult distal radius fractures did not address CTR at the time of distal radius fixation, some authors have studied the role of prophylactic CTR at the time of fixation.

Odumala and colleagues[12] retrospectively reviewed prophylactic CTR performed at the time of volar plate fixation in 69 asymptomatic patients with distal radius fractures. The first group consisted of 45 patients undergoing distal radius fixation with use of a volar Henry approach and without a concurrent CTR. The second group consisted of 24 patients who had distal radius fixation with a prophylactic CTR performed at the time of surgery. This incision also had a volar Henry approach but included an extension to the ulnar side of the thenar eminence to perform the CTR. Postoperatively, 38% (9 of 24) of patients who underwent a concurrent prophylactic CTR had median nerve dysfunction compared with 18% (8 of 45) of patients who did not receive a CTR. Most patients had spontaneous resolve of their symptoms; however, 4% in each group required further surgery for CTS. These authors thought that a prophylactic CTR at the time of distal radius fixation may lead to more complications than not performing a CTR.

Other authors have used a different incision in performing a concurrent CTR at the time of distal radius fixation. Gwathmey and colleagues[47] reviewed all adult patients during a 4-year period who had undergone an open reduction internal fixation of a distal radius fracture with a concurrent CTR. None of the patients had preoperative signs or symptoms of acute CTS related to the fracture. A chart review and telephone questionnaire were performed for all patients who met the inclusion criteria, to identify postoperative median nerve dysfunction, recurrent motor or palmar cutaneous branch injury, and tendon, injury, or other complications. Among the 65 eligible patients, 2 cases of late median neuropathy were noted. No patients required any additional surgery for early or late median nerve dysfunction. Also, no complications related to the approach, sensory or motor branch injuries, or tendon injuries were seen. Unlike other studies, which also attempted to evaluate a concurrent CTR at the time of distal radius fixation, these authors used a hybrid flexor carpi radialis (FCR) approach involving a radial-sided release of the transverse carpal ligament. This approach did not include extension of the skin incision across the wrist crease and avoided direct contact with the median nerve. Weber and Sanders noted that postoperative magnetic resonance imaging demonstrated that a radial-sided division of the transverse carpal ligament (TCL) is distant from the median nerve.[48] The lack of disruption of soft tissues in direct contact with the median nerve also may prevent perineural adhesions and preserve direct padding. Gwathmey and colleagues[47] thought that a concurrent CTR through a hybrid FCR approach could perhaps reduce the incidence of a postoperative median neuropathy, while avoiding the complications of a traditional CTR. Weaknesses of the study include its retrospective nature, potential recall bias by the patients surveyed, a lack of objective measurements, and the proportion of patients who were lost to follow-up (29 of 98 patients).

AUTHOR RECOMMENDATIONS

The presentation of CTS acutely or delayed is common following distal radius fractures, and the treating surgeon must be highly aware of this. Our recommendations include the following:

- Gross deformity of the wrist following distal radius fractures should be expeditiously reduced to mitigate the risk of median nerve injury.
- Acute CTS presenting with painful paraesthesias in the hand requires urgent decompression and fixation of the fracture.
- Prophylactic release of the carpal tunnel during fracture fixation is not recommended unless the patient has a prior history of CTS or is demonstrating active median nerve paraesthesias preoperatively.
- If a concomitant CTR is to be performed, it should be performed through a separate incision or through a radial-sided hybrid FCR approach.
- Delayed presentation of CTS following a healed distal radius fracture is best treated as an idiopathic CTS, including evaluation with electrodiagnostic testing.

SUMMARY

CTS is a common condition and is a well-recognized phenomenon following a distal radius fracture. The treating surgeon should be vigilant in noticing signs and symptoms of CTS following a distal radius fracture. If acute CTS is noted, then surgical release of the carpal tunnel and fracture fixation should be performed expeditiously. If delayed CTS is noted after distal radius fracture management, all potential causes should be evaluated for, including prominent volar cortical fragments causing direct compression of the median nerve, inadequate fracture reduction, and iatrogenic causes such as prominently placed hardware. With the current available evidence, there is no role for prophylactic CTR at the time of distal radius fixation in patients who are symptom free.

REFERENCES

1. Chung KC, Spilson SV. The frequency and epidemiology of hand and forearm fractures in the United States. J Hand Surg Am 2001;26(5):908–15.
2. Kakarlapudi TK, Santini A, Shahane SA, et al. The cost of treatment of distal radial fractures. Injury 2000;31(4):229–32.
3. Healthcare Cost and Utilization Project Nationwide Inpatient Sample, in HCUP NIS. 2007, Agency for Healthcare Research and Quality.

4. Chen NC, Jupiter JB. Management of distal radial fractures. J Bone Joint Surg Am 2007;89(9):2051–62.

5. Court-Brown CM, Caesar B. Epidemiology of adult fractures: a review. Injury 2006;37(8):691–7.

6. Wolfe S. Green's operative hand surgery. 6th edition. Philadelphia: Elsevier/Churchill Livingstone; 2010.

7. Cooney WP 3rd, Dobyns JH, Linscheid RL. Complications of Colles' fractures. J Bone Joint Surg Am 1980;62(4):613–9.

8. McCarroll HR Jr. Nerve injuries associated with wrist trauma. Orthop Clin North Am 1984;15(2):279–87.

9. Adamson JE, Srouji SJ, Horton CE, et al. The acute carpal tunnel syndrome. Plast Reconstr Surg 1971;47(4):332–6.

10. Bruske J, Niedźwiedź Z, Bednarski M, et al. Acute carpal tunnel syndrome after distal radius fractures–long term results of surgical treatment with decompression and external fixator application. Chir Narzadow Ruchu Ortop Pol 2002;67(1):47–53 [in Polish].

11. Dyer G, Lozano-Calderon S, Gannon C, et al. Predictors of acute carpal tunnel syndrome associated with fracture of the distal radius. J Hand Surg Am 2008;33(8):1309–13.

12. Odumala O, Ayekoloye C, Packer G. Prophylactic carpal tunnel decompression during buttress plating of the distal radius: is it justified? Injury 2001;32(7):577–9.

13. Abbot L, Saunders J. Injuries of the median nerve in fracture of the lower end of the radius. Surg Gynecol Obstet 1933;57:507–16.

14. Aro H, Koivunen T, Katevuo K, et al. Late compression neuropathies after Colles' fractures. Clin Orthop Relat Res 1988;233:217–25.

15. Chapman DR, Bennett JB, Bryan WJ, et al. Complications of distal radial fractures: pins and plaster treatment. J Hand Surg Am 1982;7(5):509–12.

16. Kozin SH, Wood MB. Early soft-tissue complications after fractures of the distal part of the radius. J Bone Joint Surg Am 1993;75(1):144–53.

17. Lewis MH. Median nerve decompression after Colles's fracture. J Bone Joint Surg Br 1978;60-B(2):195–6.

18. Paley D, McMurtry RY. Median nerve compression by volarly displaced fragments of the distal radius. Clin Orthop Relat Res 1987;215:139–47.

19. Szabo RM, Madison M. Carpal tunnel syndrome. Orthop Clin North Am 1992;23(1):103–9.

20. Bacorn RW, Kurtzke JF. Colles' fracture; a study of two thousand cases from the New York State Workmen's Compensation Board. J Bone Joint Surg Am 1953;35-A(3):643–58.

21. Heim D, Stricker U, Rohrer G. Carpal tunnel syndrome after trauma. Swiss Surg 2002;8(1):15–20 [in German].

22. Lidstrom A. Fractures of the distal end of the radius. A clinical and statistical study of end results. Acta Orthop Scand Suppl 1959;41:1–118.

23. Stark WA. Neural involvement in fractures of the distal radius. Orthopedics 1987;10(2):333–5.

24. Young BT, Rayan GM. Outcome following nonoperative treatment of displaced distal radius fractures in low-demand patients older than 60 years. J Hand Surg Am 2000;25(1):19–28.

25. Nishimura A, Ogura T, Hase H, et al. Evaluation of sensory function after median nerve decompression in carpal tunnel syndrome using the current perception threshold test. J Orthop Sci 2003;8(4):500–4.

26. Puchalski P, Zyluk A. Complex regional pain syndrome type 1 after fractures of the distal radius: a prospective study of the role of psychological factors. J Hand Surg Br 2005;30(6):574–80.

27. Sponsel KH, Palm ET. Carpal tunnel syndrome following Colles' fracture. Surg Gynecol Obstet 1965;121(6):1252–6.

28. Kongsholm J, Olerud C. Carpal tunnel pressure in the acute phase after Colles' fracture. Arch Orthop Trauma Surg 1986;105(3):183–6.

29. Gelberman RH, Garfin SR, Hergenroeder PT, et al. Compartment syndromes of the forearm: diagnosis and treatment. Clin Orthop Relat Res 1981;161:252–61.

30. Zachary R. Thenar palsy due to compression of the median nerve in the carpal tunnel. Surg Gynecol Obstet 1945;81:213–21.

31. Lynch AC, Lipscomb PR. The carpal tunnel syndrome and Colles' fractures. JAMA 1963;185:363–6.

32. Goldie BS, Powell JM. Bony transfixion of the median nerve following Colles' fracture. A case report. Clin Orthop Relat Res 1991;273:275–7.

33. McClain EJ, Wissinger HA. The acute carpal tunnel syndrome: nine case reports. J Trauma 1976;16(1):75–8.

34. Kinley DL, Evarts CM. Carpal tunnel syndrome due to a small displaced fragment of bone. Report of a case. Cleve Clin Q 1968;35(4):215–21.

35. Cannon BW, Love JG. Tardy median palsy; median neuritis; median thenar neuritis amenable to surgery. Surgery 1946;20:210–6.

36. Lewis D, Miller EM. Peripheral nerve injuries associated with fractures. Ann Surg 1922;76(4):528–38.

37. Watson-Jones R. Leri's pleonosteosis, carpal tunnel compression of the median nerves and Morton's metatarsalgia. J Bone Joint Surg Br 1949;31B(4):560–71.

38. Itsubo T, Hayashi M, Uchiyama S, et al. Differential onset patterns and causes of carpal tunnel syndrome after distal radius fracture: a retrospective study of 105 wrists. J Orthop Sci 2010;15(4):518–23.

39. Bienek T, Kusz D, Cielinski L. Peripheral nerve compression neuropathy after fractures of the distal radius. J Hand Surg Br 2006;31(3):256–60.

40. Gartland JJ Jr, Werley CW. Evaluation of healed Colles' fractures. J Bone Joint Surg Am 1951; 33-A(4):895–907.

41. Dresing K, Peterson T, Schmit-Neuerburg KP. Compartment pressure in the carpal tunnel in distal fractures of the radius. A prospective study. Arch Orthop Trauma Surg 1994;113(5):285–9.

42. Fuller DA, Barrett M, Marburger RK, et al. Carpal canal pressures after volar plating of distal radius fractures. J Hand Surg Br 2006;31(2):236–9.

43. Lichtman DM, Bindra RR, Boyer MI, et al. Treatment of distal radius fractures. J Am Acad Orthop Surg 2010;18(3):180–9.

44. Zollinger PE, Tuinebreijer WE, Breederveld RS, et al. Can vitamin C prevent complex regional pain syndrome in patients with wrist fractures?

A randomized, controlled, multicenter dose-response study. J Bone Joint Surg Am 2007;89(7): 1424–31.

45. Zollinger PE, Tuinebreijer WE, Kreis RW, et al. Effect of vitamin C on frequency of reflex sympathetic dystrophy in wrist fractures: a randomised trial. Lancet 1999;354(9195):2025–8.

46. Henry M, Stutz C. A prospective plan to minimise median nerve related complications associated with operatively treated distal radius fractures. Hand Surg 2007;12(3):199–204.

47. Gwathmey FW Jr, Brunton LM, Pensy RA, et al. Volar plate osteosynthesis of distal radius fractures with concurrent prophylactic carpal tunnel release using a hybrid flexor carpi radialis approach. J Hand Surg Am 2010;35(7):1082–1088.e4.

48. Weber RA, Sanders WE. Flexor carpi radialis approach for carpal tunnel release. J Hand Surg Am 1997;22(1):120–6.

Radial Tunnel Syndrome

Nash H. Naam, MD[a,*], Sajjan Nemani, MD[b]

KEYWORDS

- Radial • Tunnel • Posterior interosseous nerve • Entrapment • Neuropathy

KEY POINTS

- Radial tunnel syndrome is a pain syndrome caused by compression of the posterior interosseus nerve at the proximal forearm.
- Diagnosis depends on clinical presentation and physical findings.
- There are no specific electrodiagnostic findings.
- Conservative treatment should be tried first before resorting to surgical intervention.
- Surgical treatment is generally successful, but workers' compensation patients and those with associated lateral epicondylitis may have less successful outcomes.

INTRODUCTION

Radial tunnel syndrome (RTS) is a pain syndrome presumed to be caused by compression of the posterior interosseous nerve (PIN) at the proximal forearm. The lack of specific electrodiagnostic and pathophysiologic findings makes this syndrome somewhat controversial.[1] In 1883, Winckworth recognized the possibility of entrapment of the PIN as it passes through the substance of "supinator brevis muscle."[2] In 1966, Sharrard[3] reported the first series of patients with RTS treated surgically. In 1972, Roles and Maudsley[2] identified the association between pain and compression of the PIN, and termed the condition RTS or resisted tennis elbow.

ANATOMY

The radial tunnel is a potential space located anterior to the proximal radius through which the PIN passes. The tunnel extends for approximately 5 cm starting from the level of the humeroradial joint and extending past the proximal edge of the supinator.[4–7] The tunnel is bound on the lateral side by the brachioradialis (BR), the extensor carpi radialis longus (ECRL) and extensor carpi radialis brevis (ECRB) muscles, and on the medial side by the biceps tendon and the brachialis. Its floor is formed by the capsule of the radiocapitellar joint that extends distally to the deep head of the supinator muscle.[4–7] The radial nerve splits into the radial sensory nerve and the PIN proximal to the supinator at the elbow joint. The PIN is the motor terminal branch of the radial nerve. As the PIN crosses the elbow it passes beneath several potential compressing structures: the proximal aponeurotic edge of the supinator (also known as the arcade of Frohse); the sharp medial edge of the extensor carpi radialis brevis; the radial recurrent blood vessels; and the inferior margin of the superficial layer of the supinator muscle.[4,8–11] The arcade of Frohse is mentioned as the most frequent site of entrapment of the PIN. In a cadaveric dissection, Clavert and colleagues[10] found it to be tendinous in approximately 80% of cases. Passive stretching of the supinator muscle increases the pressure inside the radial tunnel from a normal value of 40 to 50 mm Hg to as high as 250 mm Hg.[12,13] Erak and colleagues[14] studied the radial tunnel pressure using a balloon catheter in 5 cadaveric elbows, and found that

The authors have nothing to disclose.
a Plastic and Reconstructive Surgery, Southern Illinois Hand Center, Southern Illinois University, 901 Medical Park Drive, Effingham, IL 62401, USA; b Department of Neurology, Southern Illinois Hand Center, 901 Medical Park Drive, Effingham, IL 62401, USA
* Corresponding author. 901 Medical Park Drive, Suite 100, Effingham, IL 62401.
E-mail address: drnaam@handdocs.com

orthopedic.theclinics.com

the pressure inside the radial tunnel increased when the wrist was moved from neutral to a flexion-pronation position. That increase in pressure was reduced by lengthening the supinator. Lengthening the extensor carpi radialis brevis or the extensor digitorum communis had no effect.[14]

PATHOPHYSIOLOGY

It is worth noting here that the diagnosis of RTS is doubted by several investigators, based on the fact that this syndrome is primarily a pain syndrome with no identifiable radiologic, electrodiagnostic, or pathophysiologic findings.[6,7,15–17]

One of the issues not completely understood is why an entrapment of a "purely motor nerve" could present only as a pain syndrome with no motor involvement. One explanation is that the PIN also carries unmyelinated (Group IV) and small myelinated (Group IIA) afferent fibers from the muscles along its distribution.[18] The unmyelinated Group IV fibers are called C-fibers when they are of cutaneous origin, and they have long been associated with nociception and pain. The small myelinated Group IIA afferent fibers have been associated with temperature sensation. The unmyelinated and small myelinated fibers cannot be evaluated by nerve-conduction studies. It is postulated that moderate pressure on the unmyelinated and small myelinated fibers of the PIN may produce the pain associated with the clinical presentation of RTS. The large myelinated fibers of the PIN remain essentially normal, which may explain the normal electromyography (EMG) and nerve-conduction findings.[16–23]

CLINICAL PRESENTATION

Patients with RTS usually present with pain along the dorsoradial aspect of the proximal forearm. The pain may radiate proximally and distally. The pain has a tendency to increase with rotational activities of the forearm.[7] Muscle weakness may be present with RTS on account of the pain and may not due to specific muscle dysfunction or denervation.[19] There are no sensory symptoms associated with RTS.

OCCUPATIONAL RISK FACTORS

Very few studies in the literature have examined the correlation between work activities and the incidence of RTS. A systematic literature review by Van Rijn and colleagues[24] demonstrated an increased incidence of RTS with specific work activities such as handling tools with full extension of the elbow. Roquelaure and colleagues[25] compared 21 patients with RTS with 21 volunteers,

and identified some risk factors related to work activities. It was found that regular use of a force of at least 1 kg for more than 10 times per hour with the elbow constantly extended between 0° and 45° with frequent pronation and supination of the forearm would increase the chance of developing RTS.[25]

PHYSICAL EXAMINATION

Localized focal tenderness over the anatomic landmark of the PIN is considered to be the hallmark of diagnosis of RTS.[19,26,27] The diagnosis can be difficult because of the close proximity of the site of maximum tenderness to the lateral epicondyle, which may be also involved with lateral epicondylitis. Loh and colleagues[28] proposed a novel test in which 9 equal squares are drawn on the anterior aspect of the forearm, which are then used to note where the tenderness can be elicited. Localized tenderness involving the lateral column of 3 squares was consistent with pressure over the PIN. Tenderness of RTS should be differentiated from that of lateral epicondylitis. The site of tenderness in RTS is approximately 3 to 5 cm distal to the lateral epicondyle over the supinator muscle mass. Furthermore, the pain of RTS usually does not increase by active extension of the wrist against resistance.

Patients with RTS may have weakness of their extensors. However, the weakness is mainly attributed to the pain and not to dysfunction of the extensor muscles.[19] There is no sensory deficit in patients with RTS.

Additional provocative tests have been described, including increased pain with resisted active forearm supination and pain with active extension of the middle finger against resistance.[19] The specificity and sensitivity of these tests have not been established.

Another diagnostic tool that can help to establish the clinical diagnosis, and to differentiate RTS from lateral epicondylitis, is injection of local anesthetic into the area of the localized tenderness.[20,29] However, it is important to ensure that the injected local anesthetic does not spread to the area of the lateral epicondyle.

RADIOGRAPHIC TESTING

Routine radiologic evaluation is nondiagnostic in RTS. However, magnetic resonance imaging techniques have been used to evaluate the area of the radial tunnel.[30–32] Ferdinand and colleagues[30] evaluated 10 asymptomatic volunteers and compared them with 25 patients with RTS. Fifty-two percent of RTS patients had evidence of denervation edema or atrophy within the supinator muscle or the extensor muscles innervated by the PIN. Twenty-eight percent of the patients had other findings such as thickened leading edge of the extensor carpi radialis brevis, prominent radial recurrent vessels, or schwannoma-like swelling of the nerve. The remaining patients had normal findings.[30]

ELECTRODIAGNOSTIC TESTING

One of the most challenging aspects of diagnosing RTS is the absence of standardized electrodiagnostic findings on both nerve-conduction velocity (NCV) and electromyography (EMG) studies. Frequently the electrodiagnostic studies are normal. Slowing of conduction velocity across the PIN through the supinator muscle, particularly if the testing is done at rest and with resisted supination, may be helpful.[33,34] Slowing of the conduction velocity of greater than 10 m/s or, rarely, a conduction block may be supportive of the diagnosis. Kupfer and colleagues[33] suggested modifying the standard electrodiagnostic testing to provide a more sensitive test for evaluation of RTS. These investigators recorded motor nerve latencies at 3 different forearm positions: neutral, passive supination, and passive pronation. Their findings in 25 patients with RTS with 25 asymptomatic volunteers were compared, and demonstrated that in patients with RTS there was greater differential latency versus controls. Following PIN decompression, the differential motor latencies in the test group decreased to below the control values. It was concluded that a differential motor latency of more than 0.3 millisecond is a more sensitive diagnostic tool in patients with RTS.[33]

Seror[34] used the difference in motor latency between the nerve to the BR and the nerve to the extensor carpi ulnaris as a method to diagnose RTS. EMG evidence of denervation of the PIN innervated muscles is rare.

Whereas NCV may not be helpful in establishing the diagnosis of RTS, the EMG component may have a role in its diagnosis. When EMG is positive it may be very helpful, particularly when denervation changes or abnormal motor-unit changes are seen. It is also important in ruling out concurrent cervical radiculopathy, especially at C6-C7 level, because symptoms may sometimes overlap. Overall electrodiagnostic studies may help identify associated entrapment neuropathy, and should be considered as a part of the evaluation.

However, the lack of specific electrodiagnostic findings makes the utility of electrodiagnostic testing in RTS somewhat questionable.[1]

TREATMENT

Patients with RTS should be treated conservatively before considering surgical intervention.[4,29,34] Conservative treatment, in the form of wrist splinting, activity modification, nonsteroidal anti-inflammatory medications, and possibly a therapy program may bring a resolution of patients' symptoms.[35] Patients should avoid frequent provocative maneuvers that may increase the symptoms, such as prolonged elbow extension with forearm pronation and wrist flexion. Ergonomic evaluation and education may be of value in certain situations. Modalities such as ultrasound, fluidotherapy, superficial heat, or cryotherapy have been used.[35] However, there are no studies to support the efficacy of such treatments.

Steroid injections are frequently used to help establish a diagnosis and may also have a role in conservative treatment. Sarhadi and colleagues[29] reported on 25 patients with RTS who were treated with steroid injections, and found that 18 patients (72%) improved with a single injection of 40 mg of triamcinolone and 2 mL of 1% lidocaine at 6 weeks, while 16 patients (62%) continued to be pain free for 2 years.

The effectiveness of conservative treatment has not been studied in the literature, so the optimal period of conservative treatment is not known. In general, conservative treatment is implemented for at least 3 to 6 months. Further studies into the effectiveness of conservative treatment are needed.

SURGICAL TREATMENT

If conservative treatment fails to improve patients' symptoms then surgical treatment is indicated. Surgical treatment is considered effective in general; however, many investigators suggest caution before proceeding with surgical intervention.[6,20,21,29,36–38]

Anesthesia

Regional anesthesia is adequate for RTS release. The authors prefer Bier block anesthesia, but axillary block or general anesthesia can also be used.

Surgical Technique

Several approaches have been described for the release of the RTS. The PIN can be exposed either anteriorly or dorsally.[2,5,16,19,29,36,39] Three different planes can be used through the dorsal approach. The first is between the ECRB and the extensor digitorum communis (EDC); the second is between the BR and the ECRL; and the third is a transmuscular BR-splitting approach.[5]

The authors prefer the approach between ECRB and EDC.

Dorsal (Henry) approach

The forearm is held midway between pronation and supination. The bulky muscle mass along the dorsoradial aspect of the proximal forearm, or the mobile wad, which is formed by the muscle bellies of the BR, the ECRL and ECRB is palpated, and the groove between the mobile wad and the rest of the extensor muscles is identified. An oblique incision is made along the dorsoradial aspect of the proximal forearm starting from a point about 2 cm distal to the lateral epicondyle and extending along the interval between the mobile wad and the rest of the extensor muscles (**Fig. 1**). The posterior cutaneous nerve of the forearm is usually located anterior to this incision, and should be identified and protected. A well-defined fascial interval serves as a landmark between the ECRB and the EDC (**Fig. 2**). This interval is well developed distally, and therefore it is easier if the dissection progresses from distal to proximal, separating the 2 muscles bluntly. After separation of the 2 muscles, the underlying supinator muscle, with its characteristic shiny oblique fibers, is identified (**Fig. 3**). Along the proximal edge of the supinator muscle the arcade of Frohse is identified as a tendinous band (**Fig. 4**). The PIN is located proximal to the arcade of Frohse, surrounded by some fatty tissues. The radial recurrent blood vessels (leash of Henry) are identified just proximal to the arcade of Frohse and are ligated (**Figs. 5** and **6**). The inferior margin of the supinator is also exposed. The arcade of Frohse is divided, and the superficial head of the supinator muscle is divided throughout its whole length to ensure that the inferior margin of the supinator is completely released (**Figs. 7** and **8**). The incision can be extended proximally if surgical treatment of associated lateral epicondylitis is indicated.

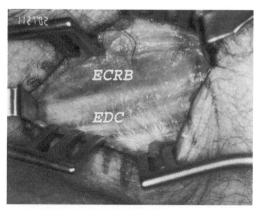

Fig. 2. The fascial interval between the extensor carpi radialis brevis (ECRB) and extensor digitorum communis (EDC) is clearly identified.

The wound is injected with bupivacaine and a soft compressive dressing is applied. Some prefer to use postoperative splinting, but generally speaking a splint is not needed.[27]

Transmuscular brachioradialis-splitting approach

The incision is slightly anterior to the incision described above. The fascia over the BR muscle is divided and the muscle fibers are split bluntly until the radial nerve is identified. The arcade of Frohse and the superficial head of the supinator muscle are divided completely.

Dorsal approach between brachioradialis and wrist extensors

The same incision or a lazy S incision can be used.[39] The interval between the BR and ECRL is identified. The posterior cutaneous nerve of the forearm is identified and protected. The fascial interval between the 2 muscles is developed. The

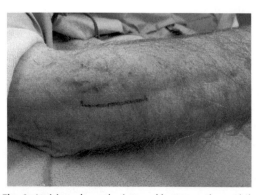

Fig. 1. Incision along the interval between the mobile wad and the rest of the extensor muscles.

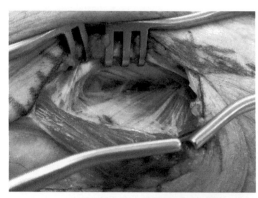

Fig. 3. The supinator muscle is identified after retraction of the ECRB and EDC. The posterior interosseous nerve (PIN) is visible along the superior edge of the supinator.

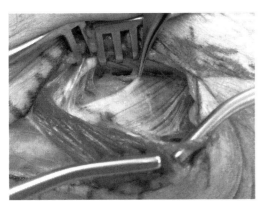

Fig. 4. The arcade of Frohse is held by a forceps along the superior edge of the supinator muscle. The PIN is identified proximal to the arcade.

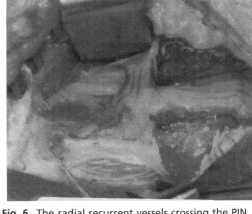

Fig. 6. The radial recurrent vessels crossing the PIN.

rest of the dissection can be continued bluntly to expose the arcade of Frohse. Some investigators advocate the release of the ECRB tendon from its origin at the lateral epicondyle as a method to treat any associated lateral epicondylitis.[5,39]

Anterior approach

In cases where there is concomitant compression of the radial nerve proximal to the elbow, the anterior approach can be very useful because it explores the radial nerve at the distal upper arm and then traces the nerve as it divides into the main terminal branches.

A curvilinear incision is made starting proximal to the lateral epicondyle and extending distally along the interval between the BR and the biceps. The incision is extended along the mobile wad and along the ulnar border of the BR. The radial nerve is identified in the interval between the BR and brachialis. The nerve is followed distally as it bifurcates into the superficial radial nerve and the PIN. The arcade of Frohse is released and the

radial recurrent blood vessels are ligated. The entire length of the supinator is visualized and completely released.

Operative Findings

Most of the time, the PIN is normal in appearance. Sometimes changes can be seen, ranging from flattening or congestion of the nerve at the level of the arcade of Frohse to a swelling and pseudoneuroma formation proximal to the arcade of Frohse (**Figs. 9–11**).

Postoperative Care

The dressing is removed 3 to 5 days postoperatively and patients are started on active range of motion. The sutures are removed in 2 weeks. Strengthening exercises are started in 3 to 4 weeks. Patients may start light duty work at 2 to 3 weeks and may resume regular work activities in 4 to 6 weeks.

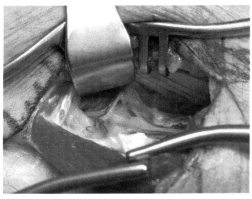

Fig. 5. The PIN is crossed by the radial recurrent vessels (leash of Henry).

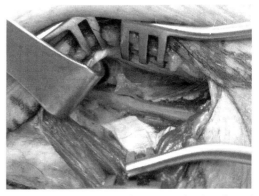

Fig. 7. The supinator has been completely released, exposing the PIN. Note the fusiform swelling of the PIN just proximal to the arcade of Frohse.

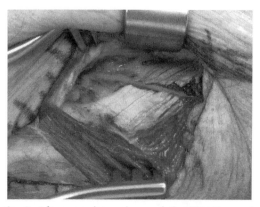

Fig. 8. After complete release of the PIN, the supinator muscle is left to return to normal position.

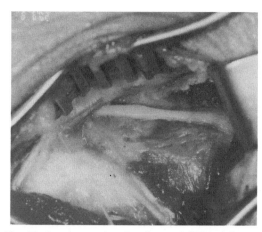

Fig. 10. Another patient in whom swelling of the PIN is identified after release of the supinator.

RESULTS OF TREATMENT

There are no available randomized controlled studies or controlled clinical trials in the literature regarding the effectiveness of conservative or surgical treatment of RTS. Huisstede and colleagues,[40] in a systematic review of observational studies, selected 6 high-quality studies out of 21 published studies. These investigators found that the effectiveness of surgical decompression ranged from 67% to 92% based on the clinical evaluation criteria established by Roles and Maudsley[2] or Loh and colleagues.[28] There is a lot of variability in the outcome of surgical treatment of RTS in the literature. For instance, Werner and colleagues[13] had a success rate of 81% following surgical decompression of RTS in 90 patients. Hagert and colleagues[26] reported 84% success in 50 patients. Lister and colleagues[19] reported pain relief in 95% of their patients. Some reports were not so optimistic about the outcome of surgical decompression of RTS.[22,41,42] De Smet and colleagues[42] had only 40% patient

satisfaction. Similarly, Atroshi and colleagues[22] reported 41% patient satisfaction after surgical treatment of 37 patients at an average follow-up of 3.5 years.

The presence of other associated conditions may influence the outcome as well. Lee and colleagues[43] reported good results in 86% of their patients when the patients had only RTS with no associated conditions. That success rate dropped to 57% in patients who had multiple entrapment neuropathies, and to 40% in patients who had concomitant lateral epicondylitis.[43]

Few studies have compared the outcome of surgical treatment of RTS in patients who were receiving workers' compensation benefits with the outcome in patients who were not receiving any.[15,21,43] Lee and colleagues[43] reported a success rate of 58% in patients receiving workers' compensation compared with 73% for patients who were not receiving it. Sotereanos and colleagues[21] demonstrated a low success rate of

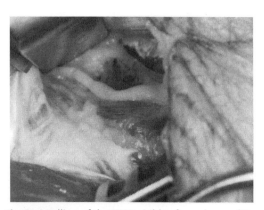

Fig. 9. Swelling of the PIN is visible after release of the supinator.

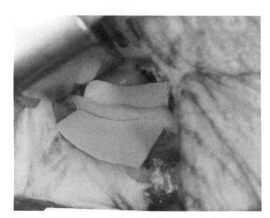

Fig. 11. Fusiform swelling of the PIN at the level of the arcade of Frohse.

32% in workers' compensation patients. Jebsen and Engber,[20] however, suggested no difference in outcome between 14 workers' compensation patients and 9 non–workers' compensation patients. However, the number of the patients in their series was relatively small, so a valid statistical analysis may not be feasible.

Patient selection for the surgical treatment of RTS is of paramount importance because the diagnostic criteria depend mainly on the clinical symptoms and physical findings. The literature supports the premise that patients with associated lateral epicondylitis and other compression neuropathies may not fare as well as patients who do not have these associated conditions. Also, workers' compensation patients have been shown to have a less successful outcome. Therefore, careful and methodical clinical evaluation is critical for the successful outcome of surgical intervention.

Despite the generally successful outcome of surgical treatment for RTS, controversy still surrounds this syndrome. Additional high-quality controlled studies are needed to evaluate the effectiveness of conservative and surgical treatment of RTS.[1,40]

REFERENCES

1. Van den Ende K, Steinmann SP. Radial tunnel syndrome. J Hand Surg Am 2010;35:1004–6.
2. Roles NC, Maudsley R. Radial tunnel syndrome: resistant tennis elbow as a nerve entrapment. J Bone Joint Surg Br 1972;54:499–508.
3. Sharrard WJ. Posterior interosseous neuritis. J Bone Joint Surg Br 1966;48:777–80.
4. Eaton CJ, Lister GD. Radial nerve compression. Hand Clin 1992;8:345–57.
5. Mackinnon SE, Novak CB. Compression neuropathies. In: Wolf SW, Hotchkiss RN, Pederson WC, et al, editors. Green's operative hand surgery. 6th edition. Philadelphia: Elsevier; 2011. p. 1005–8.
6. Rosenbaum R. Disputed radial tunnel syndrome. Muscle Nerve 1999;22:960–7.
7. Dang AC, Rodner CM. Unusual compression. Neuropathies of the forearm, part I: radial nerve. J Hand Surg Am 2009;34:1906–14.
8. Riffaud L, Morandi X, Godey B, et al. Anatomic bases for the compression and neurolysis of the deep branch of the radial nerve in the radial tunnel. Surg Radiol Anat 1999;21:229–33.
9. Portilla Molina AE, Bour C, Oberlin C, et al. The posterior interosseous nerve and the radial tunnel syndrome: an anatomical study. Int Orthop 1998; 22:102–6.
10. Clavert P, Lutz JC, Adam P, et al. Frohse's arcade is not the exclusive compression site of the radial nerve in its tunnel. Orthop Traumatol Surg Res 2009;95:114–8.
11. Konjengbam M, Elangbam J. Radial nerve in the radial tunnel: anatomic sites of entrapment neuropathy. Clin Anat 2004;17:21–5.
12. Spinner M. The arcade of Frohse and its relationship to posterior interosseous nerve paralysis. J Bone Joint Surg Br 1968;50:809–12.
13. Werner CO, Haeffner F, Rosen I. Direct recording of local pressure in the radial tunnel during passive stretch and active contraction of the supinator muscle. Arch Orthop Trauma Surg 1980;96:299–301.
14. Erak S, Day R, Wang A. The role of supinator in the pathogenesis of chronic lateral elbow pain: a biomechanical study. J Hand Surg 2004;29B:461–4.
15. Ritts GD, Wood MB, Linscheid RL. Radial tunnel syndrome. A ten-year surgical experience. Clin Orthop Relat Res 1987;201–5.
16. Steichen JB, Christensen AW. Posterior interosseous nerve compression syndrome. In: Gelberman RH, editor. Operative nerve repair and reconstruction. Philadelphia: JB Lippincott; 1991. p. 1005–22.
17. Verhaar J, Spaans F. Radial tunnel syndrome. An investigation of compression neuropathy as a possible cause. J Bone Joint Surg Am 1991;73: 539–44.
18. Lin YT, Berger RA, Berger EJ, et al. Nerve endings of the wrist joint: a preliminary report of the dorsal radiocarpal ligament. J Orthop Res 2006;24:1225–30.
19. Lister GD, Belsole RB, Kienert HE. The radial tunnel syndrome. J Hand Surg 1979;4:52–9.
20. Jebson PJ, Engber WD. Radial tunnel syndrome: long-term results of surgical decompression. J Hand Surg Am 1997;22:889–96.
21. Sotereanos DG, Varitimidis SE, Giannakopoulos PN, et al. Results of surgical treatment for radial tunnel syndrome. J Hand Surg Am 1999;24:566–70.
22. Atroshi I, Johnsson R, Ornstein E. Radial tunnel release. Unpredictable outcome in 37 consecutive cases with a 1-5 year follow-up. Acta Orthop Scand 1995;66:255–7.
23. Lawrence T, Mobbs P, Fortems Y, et al. Radial tunnel syndrome. A retrospective review of 30 decompressions of the radial nerve. J Hand Surg Br 1995;20: 454–9.
24. Van Rijn RM, Huisstede BM, Koes BW, et al. Associations between work-related factors and specific disorders at the elbow: a systematic literature review. Rheumatology 2009;48:528–36.
25. Roquelaure Y, Raimbeau G, Saint-Cast Y, et al. Occupational risk factors for radial tunnel syndrome in factory workers. Chir Main 2003;22:293–8.
26. Hagert CG, Lundborg G, Hansen T. Entrapment of the posterior interosseous nerve causing forearm pain. Scand J Plast Reconstr Surg 1977;11:205–12.
27. Barnum M, Mastey RD, Weiss AP, et al. Radial tunnel syndrome. Hand Clin 1996;12:679–89.

28. Loh YC, Lam WL, Stanley JK, et al. A new clinical test for radial tunnel syndrome—the Rule-of-Nine test: a cadaveric study. J Orthop Surg 2004;12: 83–6.

29. Sarhadi NS, Korday SN, Bainbridge LC. Radial tunnel syndrome: diagnosis and management. J Hand Surg Br 1998;23:617–9.

30. Ferdinand BD, Rosenberg ZS, Schweitzer ME, et al. MR imaging features of radial tunnel syndrome: initial experience. Radiology 2006;240:161–8.

31. Andreisek G, Crook DW, Burg D, et al. Peripheral neuropathies of the median, radial and ulnar nerves: MR imaging features. Radiographics 2006; 26:1267–87.

32. Hof JJ, Kilot M, Slimp J, et al. What's new in MRI of peripheral nerve entrapment? Neurosurg Clin N Am 2006;19:583–95.

33. Kupfer DM, Bronson J, Lee GW, et al. Differential latency testing: a more sensitive test for radial tunnel syndrome. J Hand Surg Am 1998;23:859–64.

34. Seror P. Posterior interosseous nerve conduction. A new method of evaluation. Am J Phys Med Rehabil 1996;75:35–9.

35. Cleary CK. Management of radial tunnel syndrome: a therapist's clinical perspective. J Hand Ther 2006;19:186–91.

36. Sarris IK, Papadimitriou NG, Sotereanos DG. Radial tunnel syndrome. Tech Hand Up Extrem Surg 2002; 6:209–12.

37. Stanley J. Radial tunnel syndrome: a surgeon's perspective. J Hand Ther 2006;19:180–4.

38. Kalb K, Gruber P, Landsleitner B. Compression syndrome of the radial nerve in the area of the supinator grove. Experiences with 110 patients. Handchir Mikrochir Plast Chir 1999;31:303–10.

39. Hall HC, Mackinnon SE, Gilbert RW. An approach to the posterior interosseous nerve. Plast Reconstr Surg 1984;74:435–7.

40. Huisstede BM, van Opstal T, de Ronde MT, et al. Interventions for treating radial tunnel syndrome: a systematic review of observational studies. J Hand Surg Am 2008;33:72–8.

41. Kleinert JM, Mehta S. Radial nerve entrapment. Orthop Clin North Am 1996;27:305–15.

42. De Smet L, Van Raebroeckx T, Van Ransbeeck H. Radial tunnel release and tennis elbow: disappointing results? Acta Orthop Belg 1999;65:510–3.

43. Lee JT, Azari K, Jones NF. Long term results of radial tunnel release-the effect of co-existing tennis elbow, multiple compression syndromes and workers' compensation. J Plast Reconstr Aesthet Surg 2008;61:1095–9.

Index

Note: Page numbers of article titles are in **boldface** type.

Orthop Clin N Am 43 (2012) 537–540
http://dx.doi.org/10.1016/S0030-5898(12)00099-5
0030-5898/12/$ – see front matter © 2012 Elsevier Inc. All rights reserved.

orthopedic.theclinics.com

United States Postal Service

Statement of Ownership, Management, and Circulation
(All Periodicals Publications Except Requestor Publications)

1. Publication Title	2. Publication Number	3. Filing Date
Orthopedic Clinics of North America	9 5 0 - 9 2 0	9/14/12

4. Issue Frequency	5. Number of Issues Published Annually	6. Annual Subscription Price
Jan, Apr, Jul, Oct	4	$293.00

7. Complete Mailing Address of Known Office of Publication (Not printer) (Street, city, county, state, and ZIP+4®)

Elsevier Inc.
360 Park Avenue South
New York, NY 10010-1710

Contact Person: Stephen R. Bushing

Telephone (Include area code): 215-239-3688

8. Complete Mailing Address of Headquarters or General Business Office of Publisher (Not printer)

Elsevier Inc., 360 Park Avenue South, New York, NY 10010-1710

9. Full Names and Complete Mailing Addresses of Publisher, Editor, and Managing Editor (Do not leave blank)

Publisher (Name and complete mailing address)

Kim Murphy, Elsevier, Inc., 1600 John F. Kennedy Blvd. Suite 1800, Philadelphia, PA 19103-2899

Editor (Name and complete mailing address)

David Parsons, Elsevier, Inc., 1600 John F. Kennedy Blvd. Suite 1800, Philadelphia, PA 19103-2899

Managing Editor (Name and complete mailing address)

Barbara Cohen-Kligerman, Elsevier, Inc., 1600 John F. Kennedy Blvd. Suite 1800, Philadelphia, PA 19103-2899

10. Owner (Do not leave blank. If the publication is owned by a corporation, give the name and address of the corporation immediately followed by the names and addresses of all stockholders owning or holding 1 percent or more of the total amount of stock. If not owned by a corporation, give the names and addresses of the individual owners. If owned by a partnership or other unincorporated firm, give its name and address as well as those of each individual owner. If the publication is published by a nonprofit organization, give its name and address.)

Full Name	Complete Mailing Address
Wholly owned subsidiary of	1600 John F. Kennedy Blvd., Ste. 1800
Reed/Elsevier, US holdings	Philadelphia, PA 19103-2899

11. Known Bondholders, Mortgagees, and Other Security Holders Owning or Holding 1 Percent or More of Total Amount of Bonds, Mortgages, or Other Securities. If none, check box ☑ None

Full Name	Complete Mailing Address
N/A	

12. Tax Status (For completion by nonprofit organizations authorized to mail at nonprofit rates) (Check one)
The purpose, function, and nonprofit status of this organization and the exempt status for federal income tax purposes:
☐ Has Not Changed During Preceding 12 Months
☐ Has Changed During Preceding 12 Months (Publisher must submit explanation of change with this statement)

PS Form 3526, September 2007 (Page 1 of 3 (Instructions Page 3)) PSN 7530-01-000-9931 PRIVACY NOTICE: See our Privacy policy in www.usps.com

---

13. Publication Title		14. Issue Date for Circulation Data Below
Orthopedic Clinics of North America		July 2012

15. Extent and Nature of Circulation		Average No. Copies Each Issue During Preceding 12 Months	No. Copies of Single Issue Published Nearest to Filing Date
a. Total Number of Copies (Net press run)		1245	1270
b. Paid Circulation (By Mail and Outside the Mail)	(1) Mailed Outside-County Paid Subscriptions Stated on PS Form 3541 (Include paid distribution above nominal rate, advertiser's proof copies, and exchange copies)	502	463
	(2) Mailed In-County Paid Subscriptions Stated on PS Form 3541 (Include paid distribution above nominal rate, advertiser's proof copies, and exchange copies)		
	(3) Paid Distribution Outside the Mails Including Sales Through Dealers and Carriers, Street Vendors, Counter Sales, and Other Paid Distribution Outside USPS®	420	491
	(4) Paid Distribution by Other Classes Mailed Through the USPS (e.g. First-Class Mail®)		
c. Total Paid Distribution (Sum of 15b (1), (2), (3), and (4))	▶	922	954
d. Free or Nominal Rate Distribution (By Mail and Outside the Mail)	(1) Free or Nominal Rate Outside-County Copies Included on PS Form 3541	76	99
	(2) Free or Nominal Rate In-County Copies Included on PS Form 3541		
	(3) Free or Nominal Rate Copies Mailed at Other Classes Through the USPS (e.g. First-Class Mail)		
	(4) Free or Nominal Rate Distribution Outside the Mail (Carriers or other means)		
e. Total Free or Nominal Rate Distribution (Sum of 15d (1), (2), (3) and (4))	▶	76	99
f. Total Distribution (Sum of 15c and 15e)	▶	998	1053
g. Copies not Distributed (See instructions to publishers #4 (page #3))	▶	247	217
h. Total (Sum of 15f and g)	▶	1245	1270
i. Percent Paid (15c divided by 15f times 100)		92.38%	90.60%

16. Publication of Statement of Ownership

☑ If the publication is a general publication, publication of this statement is required. Will be printed in the **October 2012** issue of this publication. ☐ Publication not required

17. Signature and Title of Editor, Publisher, Business Manager, or Owner

[signature] Stephen R. Bushing, Inventory/Distribution Coordinator

Date: September 14, 2012

I certify that all information furnished on this form is true and complete. I understand that anyone who furnishes false or misleading information on this form or who omits material or information requested on the form may be subject to criminal sanctions (including fines and imprisonment) and/or civil sanctions (including civil penalties).

PS Form 3526, September 2007 (Page 2 of 3)

Moving?

Make sure your subscription moves with you!

To notify us of your new address, find your **Clinics Account Number** (located on your mailing label above your name), and contact customer service at:

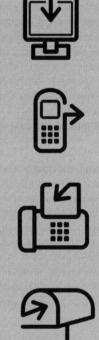

Email: journalscustomerservice-usa@elsevier.com

800-654-2452 (subscribers in the U.S. & Canada)
314-447-8871 (subscribers outside of the U.S. & Canada)

Fax number: 314-447-8029

Elsevier Health Sciences Division
Subscription Customer Service
3251 Riverport Lane
Maryland Heights, MO 63043

*To ensure uninterrupted delivery of your subscription, please notify us at least 4 weeks in advance of move.

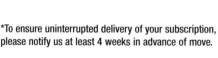
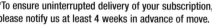

Printed and bound by CPI Group (UK) Ltd, Croydon, CR0 4YY

14/10/2024

01773652-0002